WATER: POISONED TO PURIFIED

Nullify Chemicals and Optimise Water Naturally

C Spray

Dragonwood

There are many references in this book to external sources, some of which include URLs. At the time of writing, all links were valid. However, this is the internet, and things can and do change frequently. Therefore, if you find a broken link, just search for the source document by name.

For more information, email oraphimcassie@gmail.com

ISBN: 978-1-9193409-0-6

CONTENTS

FOREWORD

My 2019 book, Shungite Reality, inspired Cassie to engage in the Shungite experience. My book is an account of my journey to understand the amazing qualities of this mineral and is an introduction to Shungite. Cassie's journey and her amazing book WATER: POISONED TO PURIFIED is a deep dive into the expanding research from many sources and her own experiences. It is a treasure of information and a must-read for anyone drawn to understand how miracles are possible with Shungite.

Nancy Hopkins

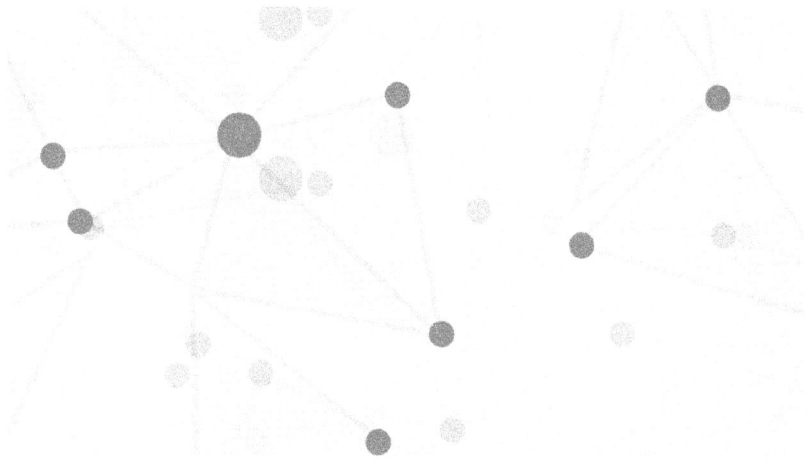

INTRODUCTION

"Our relationship with water is the most essential relationship we will have while here on planet earth."

My beautiful reader, let me ask you something profound: when did you last truly think about water? Not just "I need a drink" or "Time for a shower," but really contemplate this miraculous substance that has been your most intimate companion since before you even drew your first breath?

For nine months, you floated in perfect harmony with water in your mother's womb. You were one with it, sustained by it, cradled by it. And then? Well, then we simply got on with life, didn't we? Taking this sacred relationship completely for granted, never giving it the special attention it so deeply deserves, is something I have pondered many times. If you have picked up this book, it's reasonable for me to assume you're intrigued by it too. It's everywhere without our knowing; it's a rule-breaker, and it's unavoidable.

> *With 1 in 3 people developing cancer, we must ask:*
> *What's the one thing we all consume daily? Water.*
> *What contaminants could be making us sick?*

There are a great many people waking up to the fact that water could be—should be—so much better than what's currently flowing out of our taps. We're discovering that our municipal water, despite all those "purification" processes, arrives at our homes carrying a plethora of pollutants that would shock you if you truly understood what you've been drinking all these years.

Whether you're dealing with first-world contamination or third-world scarcity, too many of us have developed disgust and distrust, gazing upon water as the enemy instead of the life-giving miracle it was and the life-sustaining marvel it's meant to be. But beautiful you, this absolutely must change!

The Shungite Advantage: A Complete

Solution

What Shungite Delivers:
- Instant purification: Works in seconds, not hours
- Deeper detoxing and cleaning effects overall
- Energising, structuring abilities for healthy, busy lives
- Complete spectrum: Handles chemicals, bacteria, heavy metals, and toxins
- Adds beneficial frequencies: Water becomes energetically enhanced
- Never needs replacement: One purchase lasts forever
- Improves with use: Actually gets more effective over time
- Quantum intelligence: Customises its effects for each person
- No waste produced: Environmentally perfect
- No ongoing costs: No electricity, no replacement filters, no maintenance

These highlights are just the beginning of what you'll discover—I can't wait to share the complete story with you!

Falling Back In Love With Water

We can fall gently and float back into love with water. Its frequencies, its awareness of us, our continuing relationship with this divine substance—it's all deeply personal to each of us. Water's connection to us is beyond our current comprehension, but right now, in this moment, there's a new and open invitation to live happily as one with it again.

This book will guide you through making the best water

possible with Shungite solutions provided by a pioneering company called Oraphim (Oraphim mentioned in the Bible as the blueprint holders of humanity), and I promise you, we'll navigate through all the myths and misconceptions surrounding the contradictory and confusing effects that this quantum carbon mineraloid has on water. By the time we're finished, you'll understand why this ancient, mysterious gift is exactly what you and our world need right now.

Why This Follow-On Book?

My first book on this topic, "Shungite: Expect Miracles," was published in the summer of 2024 and received an astoundingly positive response. The reviews brought home to me such a profound sense of service to the growing body of literature in this magical realm of study. But as with all great publications, a revisit is always necessary!

Every book's journey is a unique blend of technical glitches, misspellings, and the inevitable evolution of understanding and ongoing revealing research. My first book was no exception. The decision to focus this revision came from others' requirements to break down the massive topic of Shungite into a mini-series of handy guides for busy lives, focusing on the key issues that matter most to you.

(Don't worry, the full immersion experience is still available in "Shungite: Expect Miracles" for those who want to dive deep!)

The Pattern Of Miracles And Shungite Effects

How do we know if something truly works? Simple: its effects are repeated over and over again. It's not a one-off miracle—it's consistently, reliably miraculous. Humans naturally seek patterns, and scientific laws are simply patterns we've learned to recognise. While some patterns are simple, others are complex. Shungite embodies both—a simple stone with complex interactions. Its behavioural patterns exist on a scale that scientists have yet to fully understand, but they're visible to those who know how to look.

Shungite creates patterns of behaviour that suggest structure, organization, and the distinct possibility of design or intelligence behind the pattern. These patterns aren't just random—they're signals, signs of communication between you and something far more profound than we initially imagined.

The trust and respect Cassie has developed for this stone and its abilities through her connection to this seemingly contradictory carbon goes beyond most Shungite research. This understanding is born from her awe and wonder at what the stone has shown her through a relationship spanning more than 25 years, beginning when she first discovered Buckminster Fuller's inspired geodesic domes in the fields of music festivals in the UK as a young woman.

Fifteen years later, she found herself standing in her own fullerene dome, working with a rule-breaking rare earth element. Remarkably, she shares the same birthday as the man it's named after—the man who discovered the natural source of the molecule that won the Nobel Prize for the very same fullerene molecule. A pattern was emerging that she could not ignore.

Dutifully, she has carried the torch for a very special Shungite compound into the lives of hundreds of thousands of people who can now benefit from it. That specially formulated compound was discovered by Nancy Hopkins. Silent internal communication *is* interaction, and Shungite is waiting to be connected with you, inviting your questions within your experience with it. You're entering into internal quantum dialogue with Shungite on a whole new level—an invitation to connect with the void, with your imagination of what can be, and all those beautiful "what if" possibilities will simply flow from you, as a stream of consciousness.

The what-ifs and the wonder at Shungite's instantaneous effects, returning the body to new heights of wellness and performance—this is utterly unique! The effect of this breaks the illusion of what we've been indoctrinated to believe about our bodies, fundamentally changing our beliefs about our entire world.

Beyond Individual Healing

It's human nature to want to do our best, isn't it? Shungite is becoming very much known for its ability to help in remarkable ways, notably for EMF protection (explored fully in the companion book 'EMF: Poisoned to Harmonised') and the purification of water. But here's where it gets exciting: Oraphim's work with Shungite has incorporated this mysterious mineraloid into a multi-stage process, pairing it with silver in ways that differ significantly from using regular stones alone.

This innovation came from Nancy L. Hopkins' groundbreaking discovery of combining these two elements, and Oraphim's work has been to develop this combination creatively in new forms, products and designs, helping get it into more people's hands who desperately need it.

What's really been needed all along is the expansion of the mind—to include this desire for being even better, even "well-er," extending beyond just yourself to share this magic and mystery that responds to you so quickly and without negative side effects. This is a revolutionary act, and you, dear reader, are part of this magnificent change.

Your Personal Revolution

When you embrace Shungite, something profound happens:
- We stop being the person with the disease
- We stop being the victim
- We stop being limited
- We stop identifying with the past or what others say about us
- We become renewed, instantly

We literally become our imagination made manifest—our vision of our very best selves. This is the world of Oraphim Shungite. This is our connection with our Creator. This is what was destined for each of us all along.

The Light Connection

Let me share something that will absolutely astound you. Mark Sloan, in his remarkable book "Red Light Therapy: Miracle Medicine," opens with this incredible statement:

"What if there was a form of therapy that could correct the root cause of virtually all diseases and conditions known to man? What if that same therapy were also inexpensive, had literally no negative side effects? Sounds too good to be true, right? I'm here to tell you this miraculous therapy does exist—it's called red and near infrared light therapy."

The fascinating thing is that Shungite naturally emits far-infrared light! I couldn't have summed up what Shungite can do for you any better than Mark did for red light therapy.

The difference? You don't need to plug Shungite in like a light bulb. You can carry it around in your pocket, and it just works amazingly well. It's like having a portable healing device that never needs charging and never stops working!

Your Invitation To Transformation

So here's my invitation to you: step into this magical world where ancient cosmic wisdom meets urgent modern need. Allow yourself to fall back in love with water. Trust in the intelligence of a unique substance that has been waiting billions of years for this moment—for you to discover its gifts and experience its transformative power.

Your relationship with water—and with your own wellbeing—is about to change forever. The patterns are about to shift. The miracles are about to begin.

Welcome to the world of Shungite water transformation. Welcome to your new relationship with the most essential element of life. Welcome to expecting miracles as your new normal.

Are you ready? Your journey has already begun.

PROLOGUE

Dear Reader,

Before I share how to transform water, I must tell you how our lives transformed—through our courage to dive into the void and allow the solutions to flow back to us when we turned away from the harmful mainstream medicine.

Oraphim was born when my partner Richard and I had let everything go. With faith and trust as our only compass, we left behind the familiar waters of conventional life. We ebbed away from our whole world—work, financial stability, communities, every aspect of modern living and the safety of known shores. Neither family nor friends became anchors holding us in place when our hearts knew the tide had turned. There was a new way planned for us all along.

We sold our tiny home—our last vestige of security—to purchase our first shipment of a rare Russian carbon. Like water finding its way through stone, we flowed into the unknown.

The void is like the space between the water molecule's

hydrogen and oxygen—seemingly empty yet holding everything together. Out of this void came our unique creative solutions, the years of pioneering research that preceded this shift, and the skills we gathered, like droplets forming a river, about to blossom into instant, transformative health tools for millions.

Seeing the implications for each development application became our daily meditation, a fluid dance of imagination and discovery. Like water taking the shape of its container, we adapted, played, explored every eddy and current of possibility. Artists do this. Inventors do this. Pioneers do this. We put all our eggs in one basket—then sold the basket to buy the egg that would hatch miracles.

Where are we now? Witnessing daily transformations as people discover what this curious, nonconforming carbon-infused water can do. Each story ripples outward, creating waves of healing.

But the topic of water goes far deeper than most realise, and we will dip into the latest discoveries, including that water's consciousness is waiting for us to remember our fluid nature. When each of us connect with our true path we can see clues laid along the way to guide us into trusting at a very deep level, for me it was the synchronicity of sharing Richard Buckminster Fuller's birthday *and* the same named towns of our birth- Milton, and with the Buckminster Fuller edition of the Times magazine published 10th January 1964, this is a quantum pairing with Richard Spray as we met in a cafe on the 10th January 2015 and he said to me, "You're not Cassie are you? I've been told I have to meet you!" These are not coincidences but confluences, streams joining a greater river.

Your soul now enters this flow. Through you, the waters of transformation rise, creating a new frequency where control and contamination cannot survive.

The invitation into water's void through Shungite is always open. It calls to souls who have quietly wondered: "What is water, really? How does Shungite reveal its mysteries?"

Let your uncertainties dissolve. Drop into not-knowing like a stone into still water. Watch the ripples of your questions expand.

What follows is not just information about purifying water, but an invitation to remember that you ARE a spirit straight from the source living in a body of water—and like water, you can transform everything you touch.

With love and anticipation for your journey, Cassie.

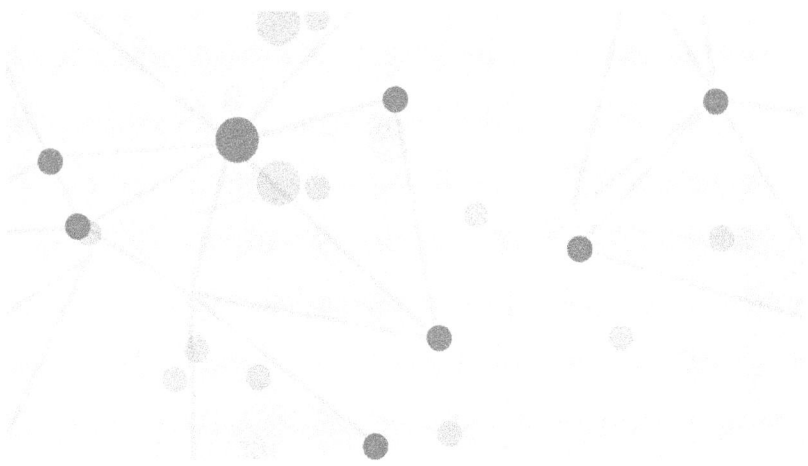

CHAPTER 1: QUICK START GUIDE

Purify Drinking Water

Contact Method 1: Simple Stone Infusion

1. Rinse 3 Shungite stones
2. Place them in a jug of water
3. Use this water for all your drinks

There is no need to wait for the purification process; it occurs instantly upon contact with the water.

Contact Method 2: Shungite Cup

1. Rinse your solid Shungite cup
2. Fill with water and drink immediately, or
3. Leave overnight for enhanced energising effects

Non-Contact Method: Oraphim Toggle
- Attach toggle to bottles, taps, garden hoses or showerheads
- Fill the glass/kettle and use water normally
- No waiting time needed—instant purification

Non-Contact Alternative Method: Charging coasters, plate or tile

- Place your jug, glass or cup on the charging coaster, plate or tile

Purify Bathing Water

Method 1: Bath Stones

Add a small collection of Shungite stones directly to bath water in a cloth bag

Method 2: Shower/Tap Toggle

Attach an Oraphim Toggle to showerheads and taps for continuous instant purification

Bonus: Replace chemical-laden commercial products with Oraphim's natural Shungite body care range for complete wellness support and electro smog removal/digital stress detox recovery

It sounds simple, but we humans love to complicate things. We measure, test, and question everything—and Shungite researchers are no different.

The problem? Many draw flawed conclusions from laboratory experiments that miss the bigger picture. Scientists design tests that produce confusing data because they haven't considered all the variables. This leads some to dismiss Shungite entirely.

At Oraphim, we think outside the test tube—literally. Our experiments revealed something remarkable: Shungite creates uniquely enhanced water tailored to each person's needs. Why? Because the experimenter affects the experiment—a quantum principle many scientists forget.
Think of it as 'quantum-infused water via divine intelligence.' Each person receives exactly the mineral frequencies their body needs in that moment.

Let's dive deeper into Shungite before tackling the most common myths about this mysterious mineraloid and emerge with a clearer understanding of this remarkable carbon.

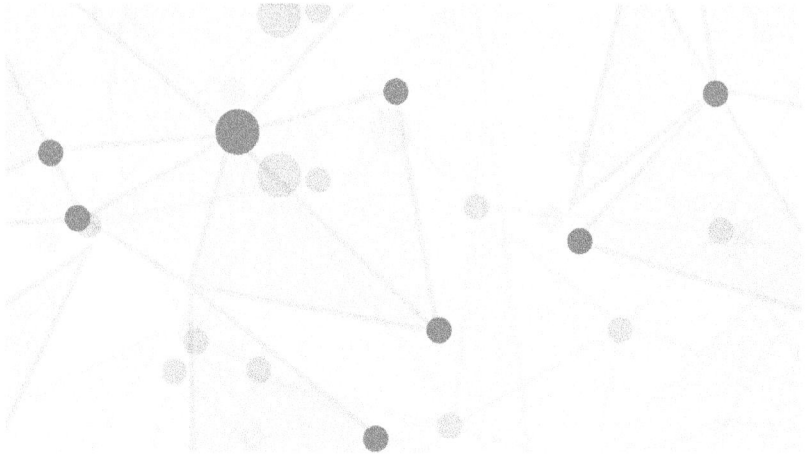

CHAPTER 2: DEEPER DIVE INTO THE UNKNOWN WORLD OF SHUNGITE

What Is Shungite? Origins And Geological Formation

Have you ever held something in your hands that completely defies everything you thought you knew about the natural world? That's Shungite—and honestly, it's about time you met this extraordinary substance that's been waiting since the beginning of time to transform your life.

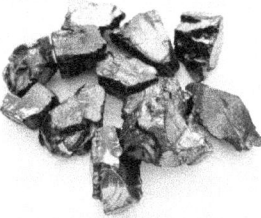

Figure 1: Shungite Stones

The Stone That Breaks All the Rules

Shungite is the rebel of the mineral kingdom. Technically, it's not even classified as a crystal (though it's commonly mistaken for one), and it can't be partnered with anything else in the carbon family—not coal, not diamonds, not graphite. Why? Because it broke their rules, too!

This remarkable carbon-based mineraloid is so unique that scientists had to create an entirely new category for it: "The Third State of Carbon." Imagine being so extraordinary that the entire scientific community has to rewrite the textbooks just to accommodate you. That's Shungite for you—completely unique, just like you are.

A Simple Test That Will Amaze You

Here's something magical you can try right now if you have a piece of Shungite: use a flat piece to scroll your phone screen, or pop a piece in the back of a torch to see it light up when the circuit is complete. Unlike coal (its closest carbon relative), Shungite offers no resistance—electrical current flows straight through it like water through an open gate.

The delight on children's faces when they make a torch flicker by wobbling a Shungite stone is absolutely priceless, and honestly, you should definitely try this at least once. It's these simple moments that reveal Shungite's extraordinary nature.

The Magnetic Mystery

Most people feel a magnetic sensation when holding Shungite stones, even though Shungite itself isn't magnetic. Try this yourself: hold a stone in each hand, place it in your fingertips, and gently move your fingertips towards and away from each other. You'll likely feel a slow bounce at about 4 to 6 inches apart—it's as if the stones are having their own little conversation, connecting through an invisible field of energy. Oraphim's work has revealed that the magnetic sensation is actually your own body's subtle electroMAGNETIC field energy.

The Land Of A Thousand Lakes

The primary source of authentic Shungite lies in Karelia, near the Finnish border with Russia—a region famously known as the "Thousand Lakes" and nicknamed "the belly of the Earth." This isn't just poetic language; it's where the earliest signs of life on our planet have been discovered, suggesting that Shungite may have been instrumental in creating the conditions for life itself.

The size of this deposit is staggering. Conservative estimates suggest it covers 621 square miles (two-thirds the size of Greater London), while others claim it spans 3,475 square miles (nearly six times the size of Greater London). With over 250 gigatons of Shungite estimated in total reserve, this remarkable substance is definitely not running out anytime soon—despite what you might hear about its scarcity.

The Greatest Geological Mystery

After more than a century of study by brilliant Russian and Western scientists, Shungite's origins remain one of the greatest puzzles of our planet. No consensus has been reached because, quite simply, Shungite doesn't fit any established rules for how things are supposed to form on Earth.

Here's what makes it so mysterious: True Shungite is found only in one place, on the border between Finland and Russia. The key to getting the correct grade is to buy Shungite from the Zazhoginsky deposit.
Shungite takes its name from the village of Shunga. Remarkably, it contains every element on the periodic table except the radioactive ones. Even more astounding, it harbours two elements rarely found on Earth: helium-3 (typically found only in space or meteorite sites) and fullerenes (associated with rare electrical phenomena).

These discoveries fuel the meteorite theory of Shungite's origins. However, my personal collection includes an elite specimen that tells a different story. Its centre clearly shows where molten material flowed out and cooled— like a liquid chocolate centre that leaked and solidified. This suggests Shungite cooled slowly from a liquid state, challenging the space-origin theory.

Theories That Spark The Imagination

The Cosmic Visitor Theory
Some researchers, including Professor Kovalevsky, believe Shungite arrived via an ancient meteor impact 2.5 billion years ago. His microscopic photographs reveal interplanetary dust particles in the samples—compelling evidence of cosmic origins. Nancy Hopkins champions this theory, explaining: "Somewhere in the cosmic landscape between the stars, carbon atoms assembled into molecules. Wherever this cosmic birthplace existed, it contained the basic building blocks of matter—especially carbon."

Regina Martino and Jessica Mahler propose an earthly origin. According to Martino: 'Shungite formed from organisms living at the beginning of the Proterozoic aeon with these unicellular prokaryotes accumulating with mud and silt, creating sedimentary layers in brackish lagoons near volcanic rifts' concluding that .'Through compression over aeons, these organic sediments transformed into rock.'

The Lost Planet Theory
This theory, championed by Shungite Healing facilitator Jarome Priest of Sacred Sounds, based in Glastonbury (UK), is the most intriguing, suggesting that Shungite could be remnants of Phaeton, a hypothetical planet that once existed between Mars and Jupiter, whose destruction supposedly created our asteroid belt.

Although these origin stories are fascinating and awe-inspiring, none of the theories adequately explain the formation of Shungite into nine distinct layers or fully answer questions about the two distinct rock-forming types within its deposit. Then there's the distinct layering within the stones themselves, including the molten core elite samples found by Cassie, and the unique fact that the deposit contains every element on the periodic table (except radioactive isotopes). This includes the extraterrestrial elements helium-3 and fullerenes, all combined together into this one outstanding rock.

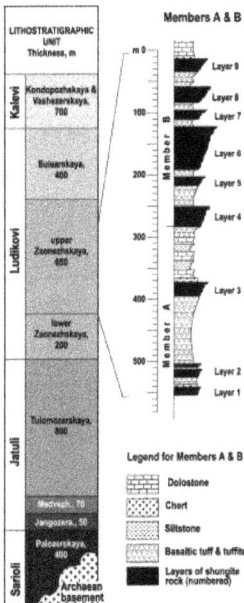

Figure 2: The Nine Layers

The Genesis Stone Theory

Published by Chris Campbell, this is my favourite, with expert insight from Dr Yuri Klavdievich, a Doctor of Technical Sciences, proposing something even more extraordinary. He suggests Shungite could have formed at the very beginning of our planet's creation, given the extremely high temperatures required to create its unique fullerene structures. As Yuri wonderfully puts it: "Shungite form emerged before other rocks and layers, the question is —may it be possible for Shungite to form at the same time as the planet Earth?"

The structure of the Shungite deposit defies simple explanations. Nine distinct layers extend 400-600 feet deep, with Elite veins just 18 inches wide running through them. This isn't one continuous mass—it's nine separate formations.

This layered structure challenges both major theories. A single meteorite couldn't create nine distinct layers. Sedimentary deposits from decaying matter wouldn't form this pattern either.

My conclusion? We're missing something extraordinary. The truth requires more open minds and wilder possibilities than current science offers. Until we discover what really happened, the ancient tales of Shungite's origins may hold more wisdom than modern theories.

Indigenous Wisdom Vs. Scientific Theory

The Keepers of Ancient Truth

While modern scientists scratch their heads and frantically revise their theories, there's another source of knowledge that has remained remarkably consistent for thousands of years: the wisdom of indigenous peoples who have lived alongside Shungite since time immemorial.

Fundamental truths travel through time as tales. Ancient peoples wove complex concepts into stories, embedding wisdom in symbols for future generations to decode. Around flickering firesides, they shared the bedtime story of Giant Valit—a being of immeasurable strength who hurled down from space a rock with 'spinning eyes.' These tales speak to our unconscious intelligence, whispering truths from the depths of the void.

The Pattern We Keep Ignoring

Isn't it fascinating how often indigenous folklore aligns more accurately with reality than scientific theory? Time and again, we see ancient wisdom validated by modern discoveries, yet the academic world continues to dismiss traditional knowledge as "primitive superstition."

But here's what gives me absolute chills: the folklore surrounding Shungite aligns with observable facts far more accurately than modern scientists would ever admit!

Why Indigenous Knowledge Matters: These ancient peoples witnessed events, experienced phenomena, and preserved memories that stretch back far beyond written history. They weren't constrained by academic theories or professional reputations. They simply told their truth as they knew it; they are cosmically connected to their environment before the distractions of any 9 to 5 modern slavery jobs or distracting technology. Knowledge was passed down to them by their ancestors.

Their Sacred Truth

"The indigenous origin story, preserved through countless generations, tells of a flying giant named Valit who hurled a space rock with 'spinning eyes' down to Earth. To me, this name speaks in quantum language—'Valit' becomes 'VITAL,' revealing why this stone matters now. As they say, it's all in the name.

The Magic of Nine Layers of Mystery: Shungite's formation

adds to its enigma: nine distinct layers spanning 400-600 feet deep. This isn't random geology—it's organised, structured, as if deliberately laid down over time. Nothing else on Earth forms this way.

The pattern mirrors how Earth energies regenerate through alternating organic and inorganic layers—what Wilhelm Reich called 'Orgone' processing. We're looking at ancient, planetary purification technology that science only recently recognised.

The Fullerene Connection: Here's where it gets extraordinary. Shungite contains fullerenes—those perfect soccer-ball carbon molecules. Science 'discovered' them in 1985, yet they've been spinning in Shungite since before the Sami told their bedtime stories.

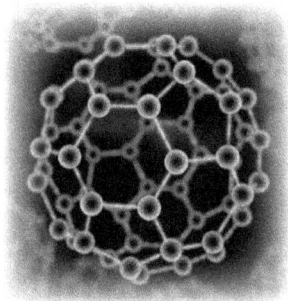

Figure 3: Fullerene

Even more remarkable? Artists knew these shapes centuries ago:
- Leonardo da Vinci drew them (1452)
- Verona carpenters carved them (1494)
- Lorenzo Sirgatti illustrated them (1596)
- Reiss Kunst depicted them (1625)
- Later called Goldberg's Polyhedra
- Richard Buckminster Fuller made them into

functioning buildings on a grand scale (1950)

Buckminster Fuller—the 'father of fullerenes'—made them famous with his geodesic domes. Those very structures inspired me to start building my own.

Using the Hubble Space Telescope, scientists have discovered that these Goldberg Polyhedra/fullerenes are abundant in space but rare on Earth, and are found mainly at meteor impact sites, lightning strikes, or other electrical phenomena. This cosmic connection adds a deeper layer to Shungite's mystery and magnificence.

The Karelia Event

On February 21, 2020, something happened that made even the most sceptical scientists sit up and take notice. A luminous blue sphere descended from the heavens and exploded directly above the Karelia Shungite deposits. This wasn't some grainy, questionable footage. It was captured on CCTV, witnessed by locals, and occurred exactly ten days before the world went into lockdown.

Coincidence? I think not.

Here's where it gets even more extraordinary. Researcher Walt Silva had been measuring Shungite's frequency for years. After this blue celestial visitor arrived? The readings shot up to an astounding 1298 GHz—a transformation so dramatic it's like your gentle house cat suddenly roaring like a lion.

What does this mean for your water? Everything. Higher frequencies enhance water's ability to restructure molecules. It's as if Shungite received a cosmic upgrade, becoming even more powerful at creating the pure, life-giving water our bodies desperately need in these challenging times.

The Hopi prophecy of the Blue Star Kachina speaks of a time of purification and transformation. Sound familiar? This isn't just some vague prediction—it's specifically about a blue celestial object that would herald a new era of cleansing.

Nancy L. Hopkins, through her remote-viewing sessions, explored the origins of this phenomenon. What she discovered adds yet another layer to Shungite's mystery —suggesting this wasn't random, but perhaps a perfectly timed gift for humanity's greatest need.

Think about it: An ancient purification stone receives a cosmic enhancement just as our world faces unprecedented challenges. The water in your glass isn't just H2O anymore—it's been touched by something that bridges Earth and stars, ancient wisdom and cutting-edge science.

From Common To Elite

Shungite comes in several beautiful varieties. Common Shungite appears as grey to black stones containing 30-64% carbon, while the rarer "Elite" stones shine with a silvery, metallic lustre and contain 98% carbon. Both share the same inherent properties—biofield enhancement, electromagnetic harmonisation, and powerful purification abilities—but each offers its own unique energy signature.

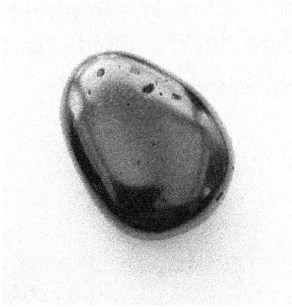

Figure 4: Elite Shungite

The darker black stones are actually more desirable for many applications, and as you'll discover throughout this book, the most expensive stones aren't always necessary for extraordinary results. Sometimes the humble black Shungite outperforms its pricier Elite cousin in ways that will surprise you.

A Bridge Between Worlds

We embarked on this journey to explore Shungite's water-transforming abilities. Remember that you're connecting with something truly special—a substance that bridges the cosmic and terrestrial, the ancient and cutting-edge, the mysterious and scientifically validated.

Shungite has puzzled scientists, healed the sick, and defied classification for centuries. It's a rule breaker. From Peter the Great's 18th-century healing spas to modern EMF protection devices, this remarkable substance continues to demonstrate abilities that place it in a category entirely its own.

What you're about to discover will transform not just your water, but quite possibly your entire understanding of what's possible when science meets the miraculous. Because with Shungite, as you'll soon learn, expecting miracles isn't just hope—it's simply good science.

Your Journey Begins

You've been guided to this knowledge for a reason. Whether you're seeking better health, cleaner water, or simply answers to questions you didn't even know you had, Shungite has been waiting for you to discover it at this moment—for you to experience its gifts and share its transformative power.

So take a deep breath, open your heart to possibility, and prepare to meet the most extraordinary molecule our planet has to offer. Once you have this knowledge, the misleading viral videos will be blasted out of the water by your own deep understanding, and nothing will get in the way of your true transformation, which has already begun, by the way.

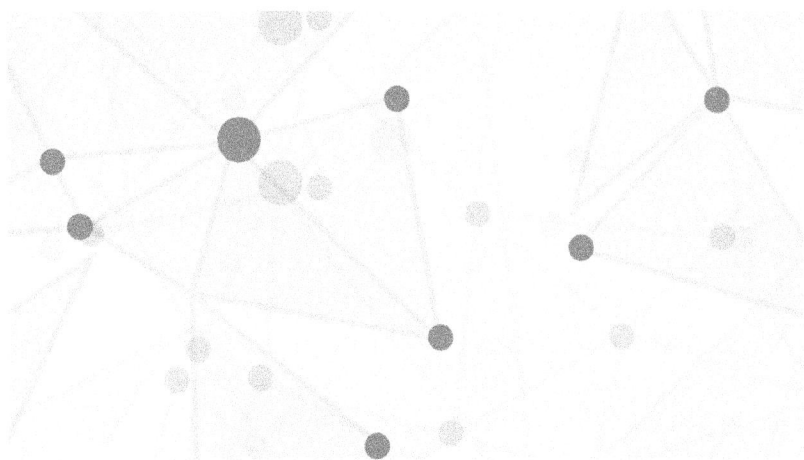

CHAPTER 3: THE FASCINATING SCIENCE OF FULLERENES IN WATER

"One of the most spiritual experiences any of us in the original team of five has ever experienced."

— *Richard Smalley, Fullerenes C60 Nobel Prize winner*

C an you imagine discovering something so profound that a Nobel Prize-winning scientist describes it as one of his most spiritual experiences? That's the power of fullerenes, you're about to understand why these tiny spinning miracles are absolutely revolutionising everything we thought we knew about water, healing, and life itself.

C60 And C70 Fullerene Structures And Properties

The Perfect Sacred Geometry

Picture this: a soccer ball so perfectly designed that it contains the secrets of the universe. That's essentially what a C60 fullerene is—a truncated icosahedron made up of 20 hexagons and 12 pentagons, creating the most stable atomic structure known to science. It's sacred geometry made manifest in carbon!

Now, here's where it gets absolutely mind-blowing: this "fullerene" shape was actually depicted by artists hundreds of years ago, long before modern science even knew these molecules existed. Leonardo Da Vinci himself sketched these very structures in the 1400s! It's as if the universe was whispering its secrets through artists long before scientists were ready to listen. 15 years before finding Shungite, Cassie was building structures based on fullerene geometry, and Susie was learning about C60 in the Cosmic

Trigger Books. Now, together with Richard, they work to produce Nancy's special silver-activated Shungite Body Care, providing natural healing and detox products for people.

The Molecular Miracle Workers

These aren't just pretty shapes. Fullerenes are molecular miracle workers with properties that seem to defy everything we thought we knew about matter.

C60 Fullerenes: These perfect spheres contain 60 carbon atoms arranged in that divine soccer ball pattern. They're like tiny, hollow cages with a vacuum inside that literally pulls toxins in while the outside attracts free radicals. Imagine having a microscopic cleaning crew working at the cellular level!

C70 Fullerenes: These are slightly larger, rugby ball-shaped molecules with 70 carbon atoms. While they're found more commonly in Elite Shungite, here's something that might surprise you: research shows that C60 molecules found in cheaper black Shungite actually have superior electromagnetic properties due to their perfect spherical shape. Sometimes the humble beats the fancy!

Speedy Transformations

The fastest molecule recorded is our very own fullerene, spinning at 20-30 billion times per second in one direction. It cannot be reversed or slowed down—in fact, its frequency is getting higher every day. It has a force far greater than one molecule spinning on its own, and this is because it was discovered to be in quantum entanglement with every other fullerene molecule. What happens to one happens to them all, wherever they are on the planet or in your pocket!

The Size That Changes Everything

Now, pay attention to this because it's absolutely crucial: fullerenes are exactly the right size to fit into the nooks and crannies of your DNA and RNA. Think of them as molecular scaffolding, perfectly designed to support the rebuilding, regeneration and activation of your cells. Think of each particle of Shungite as a portal accessing energy and delivering healing far infrared from the quantum realm.

Coincidence? I think not! It's as if they were specifically designed to heal and restore human life, but there's more to come: Activation.

Director of Science and Doctor of Philosophy, Professor G. V. Andrievsky, is the modern father of fullerene research today. He has pioneered the isolation of the true fullerenes found in Shungite. This base fluid is called "The Andrievsky Solution." His research concluded that this compound defied pharmacological classification because it acted at a systemic level, essentially correcting issues at both the cellular and whole-body levels.

He has published more than 55 groundbreaking research papers detailing the curative and healing abilities of this unique molecule. Currently working at the Institute of Physiologically Active Compounds, his research covers medicinal chemistry, nano biochemistry, and nanotechnology. His team's work was included in the international symposium on fullerenes and fullerene-like structures.

Andrievsky's conclusions about Shungite:
- 30x more powerful than activated charcoal
- Normalises cellular metabolism

- Increases enzymatic activity
- Stimulates tissue regeneration
- Increases cellular resistance
- Possesses anti-inflammatory abilities
- Fosters exchange of neurotransmitters
- Neutralises toxins, specifically supporting liver detox and function in cancer patients
- Removes necrotic cells for rapid healing

His research concluded that these fullerenes—found only in Shungite—positively affect biomolecules exposed to excess heat. They are protected by modifications to the body's proteins, which stabilise all living things. (5G is technology that, in simple terms, microwaves the cells, causing them to heat up.)

The Indestructible Healers

Here's something that will absolutely astound you: fullerenes are 30 times more effective than activated charcoal at neutralising free radicals, and unlike other antioxidants that can actually cause harm if you take too much, fullerenes remain completely safe even at concentrations 10,000 times higher than normal doses.

You literally cannot overdose on Shungite's healing power—how's that for divine design?

How Fullerenes Interact With Water Molecules

The Quantum Water Dance

When fullerenes meet water, something truly magical happens. It's not just a simple chemical reaction—it's a quantum dance between ancient cosmic intelligence and the essence of life itself.

The Hydrogen Connection

Dr Adam D. Wexler's research reveals that there are 100 sextillion drops of water in the average human body, with special positively charged hydrogen particles "crowd surfing" at supersonic speeds, searching for connection with others.

This highlights our fundamental need for connection—not just with each other, but at the molecular level. We are literally made of water that longs to connect, and Shungite facilitates these connections in the most perfect way. Shungite is reported to create hydrogen-rich water.

The Instant Transformation

Unlike traditional water treatments that slowly filter or process water, fullerenes work through what's called the "kinetic electric effect"—instant transformation at the molecular level. The moment Shungite encounters water, its sacred work begins:
- Surface tension drops instantly, allowing for proper cellular hydration
- Molecular memory gets cleared and reprogrammed with beneficial frequencies
- Toxins get neutralised rather than just filtered out
- Life force energy gets infused into every single molecule

The Ion Exchange Miracle

Here's where fullerenes show their true intelligence: they perform what I call a "divine ion exchange." Your essential minerals stay safely in your cells where they belong, while 'spent' heavy metals and damaging toxins get safely escorted out through your urine.

Free radicals typically require detox protocols for removal. Fullerenes in Shungite work differently—they intelligently donate or remove electrons based on what each free radical needs. Instead of simply eliminating these molecules, fullerenes repurpose them into useful compounds for the body. It's molecular recycling at its most sustainable level.

It's like having the most sophisticated, loving security system for your body—keeping the good stuff in and showing the harmful elements the door.

Spin Rates (20-30 Billion RPS) and Quantum Effects

Are you ready for this? Fullerenes have been measured spinning at 20-30 billion times per second—making them the fastest spinning molecules ever recorded! And here's the crucial part: they spin to the right, which is the direction of expansion, enhancement, and life force energy.

As Nancy L Hopkins so beautifully explains: "Proto-energy is pulsed into the C60 shape, spinning the molecule at 20 billion times a second. That spinning causes an energy field of extreme stability and force to exist."

Opening Doors to Other Dimensions

Now, this is where science meets the mystical in the most magical way. Torsion field physics tells us that the faster something spins, the greater its ability to access what scientists call "hyper-dimensions"—realms of energy and information beyond our ordinary three-dimensional world.

Frank, an independent inventor, discovered that due to these incredible spin speeds, fullerenes can access every frequency. This is why Shungite can deliver its unique mineral-balancing action to each cell in your body—it's literally connecting to Karelia's main Shungite deposit to bring you exactly what you need!

The Quantum Field Connection

Nancy L Hopkins puts it perfectly: "The C60 is a finite object linked to the infinite power of the quantum field." These spinning fullerenes are opening and closing doorways to the quantum realm approximately 20-30 billion times every second, allowing healing energy and information to flow from the infinite into your finite, beautiful body.

Creating Your Personal Quantum Bubble

When you work with Shungite, these spinning fullerenes create what I like to call your personal "quantum bubble"— a protective, enhancing field around you that's spinning at cosmic speeds. This is why people often describe feeling like their "wings are opening" or experiencing a gentle "whoosh" of new energy when they first encounter Shungite.

You're literally being lifted into a higher frequency state —every cell in your body receiving a faster spin rate that matches this cosmic dance!

Scientific Studies On Fullerene Water Interactions

The Evidence Keeps Pouring In

While the mainstream often tries to dismiss natural healing solutions, the scientific evidence for fullerenes and Shungite keeps mounting like a beautiful, unstoppable wave of truth.

The Medical Breakthroughs

The National Institute of Health has published studies showing that fullerenes have:
- Anti-inflammatory properties that rival pharmaceutical drugs
- Antiviral capabilities that work against multiple viral strains
- Antioxidant power that surpasses anything previously known
- Anti-HIV properties that inhibit viral replication
- Anti-venom with prophylactic abilities

The Water Purification Proof

Studies by Oleg Mosin of Moscow State University and Ignat Ignatov of Bulgaria reported remarkable findings on Shungite's water-purification abilities. They documented removal rates that will astound you:
- Iron removal: 95%
- Lead removal: 85%
 - Copper removal: 85%
- Radioactive strontium: 97%
- Harmful fluorine compounds: 80%
- Chlorine and organochlorine: 95%
- Dioxins: 97%

But here's what the studies don't fully capture: Shungite doesn't just remove these harmful elements—it transforms them at the quantum level, breaking their molecular bonds and rendering them harmless. Money-Saving Tip: Unlike traditional carbon filters that need constant replacement, Shungite offers a revolutionary solution—buy once, use forever. This unique carbon element purifies water continuously without losing effectiveness or requiring replacements.

The Cellular Studies

Recent research published in PubMed (February 2023) by Seda Beyaz and her team showed that C60 fullerene nanoparticles were effective in treating heart inflammation in rats, concluding they're "a promising and potentially effective therapy for the treatment of heart diseases associated with inflammation in humans."

This is particularly crucial given the heart inflammation issues, sadly, we're seeing more frequently these days, such as peri and myocarditis that have been linked to the experimental MRNA treatments. Once again, nature provides the solution exactly when we need it most.

The Quantum Water Analysis

Our own water analysis using the Palintest Photometer 7500 revealed something that left even us speechless: Shungite worked instantly, whether it touched the water or not. We placed toggles and stickers on the outside of test tubes, and the water remained crystal clear for five days. When the Shungite's quantum field energy dissipated, the bonds reformed, proving that molecular transformation had indeed occurred.

This isn't just filtration—it's quantum purification at the molecular level.

The Shape Memory Research

The National Institute of Health published fascinating research showing that fullerenes not only absorb electromagnetic energy but also reinforce nanoscale structures. They found that incorporating fullerenes increased the strength of materials by more than ten times.

Imagine what this means for your cellular structures! These aren't just protective molecules—they're rebuilding and strengthening your very foundation from the Inside Out.

The Homoeopathic Studies

Shungite has been successfully tested using homoeopathic approaches, in which the Shungite frequency was captured and used instead of direct contact. The results showed activation of 'KELEA'—the life energy force that various cultures call chi, prana, or orgone.

This proves that Shungite's effects aren't just physical— they're energetic, spiritual, and deeply connected to the life force itself.

The Living Proof

But perhaps the most powerful evidence isn't in laboratories—it's in the countless testimonials from people whose lives have been transformed. From thyroid conditions reversing after decades, to ganglions disappearing in hours, to respiratory conditions clearing in days, the evidence is literally walking around, breathing better, and living fuller lives.

Your Personal Laboratory

As you begin your journey with Shungite, remember that you are conducting the most important research of all —the study of your own transformation. Every glass of Shungite water you drink, every moment you spend in its quantum field, you're participating in the most beautiful experiment: the restoration of your divine blueprint.

The fullerenes spinning billions of times per second in your Shungite aren't just molecules—they're messengers from the quantum realm, carrying healing frequencies that your cells remember from the very beginning of creation.

Trust the process, document your experiences, and prepare to be amazed by what these tiny cosmic dancers can do for your life.

Natural Versus Synthetic Fullerenes: The Crucial Difference

The fascinating topic of fullerenes leads many people down an intriguing path. Since fullerenes are supposedly the fantastic driving force for purification found in Shungite, some are naturally tempted by the ability to purchase synthesised C60 fullerenes and ingest them when suspended in oil. But here's where things get absolutely fascinating—and why Mother Nature's design is always superior to our laboratory attempts to replicate it.

We at Oraphim were curious about this ourselves, so we obtained 99.9% synthesised C60 fullerenes and decided to compare them with regular Shungite, Elite Shungite, and our silver-infused Shungite using simple dowsing and strength-testing methods.

The results absolutely shocked us! The synthesised fullerenes actually drained the participant of energy and did not strengthen their energy field at all during muscle testing. Even when we infused these synthetic C60s with silver, they did not perform in the positive, life-enhancing way that silver-infused Shungite does.

In a comparison test conducted by Regina Martino, she also concluded that synthetic fullerenes resulted in a 55% loss of a person's vital energy field.

This discovery reinforced something profound: Shungite really is the most curious carbon, and there's something irreplaceably special about fullerenes that have been spinning in the Earth, awaiting their divine task to work with us versus those created in a laboratory.

Now you have some insights into this miracle-working stone; in the next chapter, we will bust the myths around this mineraloid.

So take a deeper breath, open your heart to possibility, and prepare to meet the most extraordinary molecule our planet has to offer. Once you have this knowledge, the misleading viral videos will be blasted out of the water by your own deep understanding, and nothing will get in the way of your true transformation, which has already begun, by the way.

You now have more information about this rule-breaking, non-conforming carbon than most people on the planet. Together, we will sail through the most commonly cited mistruths and misunderstandings. You will see its quantum adaptogenic nature that others have missed due to its confusing contradictions, and clearly understand why it simply works—methodically, mysteriously, and magically. Lastly, you will want to say with all your heart that Shungite is yours.

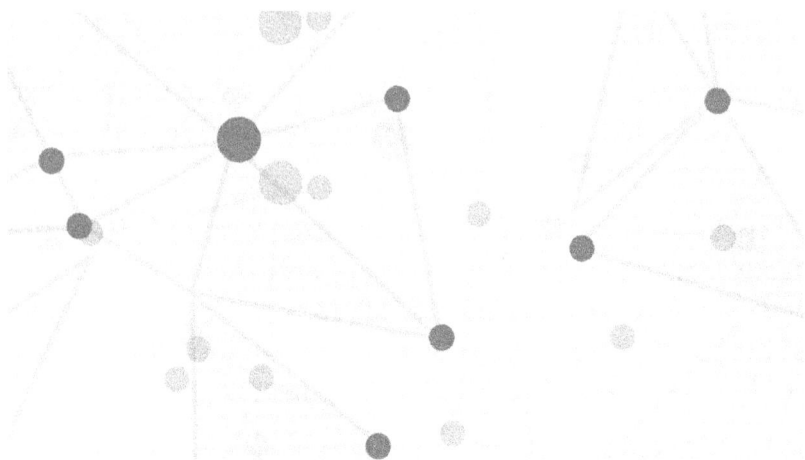

CHAPTER 4: DISPELLING THE COMMON MYTHS ABOUT SHUNGITE

"Shungite is something incomprehensible."
— Yuri Klavdievich, Russian scientist

T ruth Seekers, the misinformation floating around about this remarkable substance would be hilarious if it weren't preventing people from experiencing its life-changing benefits. Remember, ChatGPT can only scurry around and gather an overview, and it cannot discern truth from quantum actions.

Let's roll up our sleeves and tackle these myths head-on. Once you understand Shungite's true quantum abilities, you'll see why even well-meaning video makers get confused. They care about helping people, but miss the vital lesson: Shungite is personal and unique. It provides exactly what YOU need, exactly when you need it.

Myth 1: Elite Shungite Superiority

"You must use the most expensive Elite Shungite for the best results"

More Expensive Shungite Doesn't Always Mean Better

Oh, how this myth makes my heart ache! Many people spend money on Elite Shungite, believing it's superior for everything. The truth? Humble black Shungite often outperforms its expensive cousin in remarkable ways. We've witnessed life-saving transformations using common black Shungite—proof that miracles don't require the premium price tag. These stories are coming up later in the book.

The Carbon Content Reality Check

Yes, it's true that Elite Shungite contains 98% carbon compared to black Shungite's 30-64%, but here's what the sellers don't tell you: higher carbon content doesn't automatically mean better performance for every application.

The Water Purification Truth

When it comes to water purification, healing, and detoxing, you absolutely don't need to purchase the most expensive Elite Shungite stones. The cheaper grade of black Shungite will do the job effectively.

Our water analysis results prove that even a pinch of common black Shungite outperforms a 15-stage filter. If you're on a budget, don't feel you're getting second best with black Shungite. You're getting something extraordinary.

The Healing Power Stories

Let me share something that will absolutely astound you: the first life-saving transformation we witnessed involved a gentleman diagnosed with brain tumours behind each eye, given three months to live. We gave him black Shungite stones for his drinking water and a laminated patch of powder for his hat.

After accidentally receiving double the radiation dose, his liver and kidney function tests came back completely normal (which normally takes 2-3 months, but happened instantly). His tumours shrank, and his life expectancy increased to four years. This miraculous result happened with humble black Shungite, not Elite!

The Cost-Benefit Reality

Elite stones work faster by mere seconds, not hours or days. For practical water purification, the price difference simply isn't justified by the minimal performance difference. Your budget is better spent on getting more black Shungite for your whole family than on a tiny piece of Elite for just yourself.

Trust Your Intuition

If you feel drawn to Elite Shungite for personal reasons, absolutely trust that calling! But don't let anyone convince you that black Shungite is somehow "second class." or does not work. Both are integrated parts of the whole quantum fabric, and both will provide you with remarkable benefits.

The EMF Protection Surprise

Research has demonstrated that black Shungite (grade 2) is actually superior for electromagnetic devices! The magnetoresistance ratio in black Shungite C60 is approximately one order of magnitude larger than that of Elite C70-based devices at room temperature.

Nancy L Hopkins, our Wi-Fi warfare expert, recommends black Shungite that's been saturated with silver for EMF harmonisation because it simply works better. Sometimes David beats Goliath!

EMF protection is explored fully in the companion book 'EMF: Poisoned to Harmonised'.

Myth 2: 3-5 Day Purification Timeline

"It takes 3-5 days for Shungite to purify water properly"

The Instant Miracle Reality

This myth drives me absolutely bonkers because it's preventing people from experiencing Shungite's most remarkable quality: instant transformation! The idea that you need to wait days for Shungite to work is like saying you need to wait for the sun to warm your face. Nonsense!

The Molecular Bond Breaking Magic

Here's what's really happening at the quantum level: inside Shungite, there is a molecule called a fullerene spinning at 20-30 billion times per second, and these are creating a force so powerful that the chemical bonds are broken instantly—so the Shungite is never absorbing toxins, but literally breaking them apart at the molecular level.

Our Chlorine Nullification Breakthrough

Using our professional water analysis equipment, we captured something extraordinary through our testing. We tested tap water that turned yellow from a chlorine reaction with potassium iodide, but when we tested Shungite-treated water, we got instant, crystal clear results!

The transformation happened instantly, and the results showed up in the time it takes to make a cup of tea. Not hours, not days—seconds!

The 3-Day Experience

Shungite purifies water instantly—you can drink it right away. However, leaving stones in water for up to three days enhances both taste and energy.

Different Contaminants, Same Speed

Whether it's chlorine, fluoride, heavy metals, or bacteria,

Shungite's quantum action works at incredible speeds. Our fluoride experiments showed immediate results—the contaminated tap water turned orange (indicating fluoride presence), while Shungite water remained the reddest, the best result for fluoride nullification in water.

Here's something that will make you smile: Shungite-bristle toothbrushes kill harmful bacteria on contact. The moment these special bristles touch your teeth and gums, they stop bacteria dead in their tracks—no more plaque buildup, no more bacterial film. It works instantly for both humans and pets! (And yes, if you're wondering, Oraphim does supply these remarkable toothbrushes.)

David reported: "Day 3 of using your toothbrush on Jai (David's dog), and somehow I feel a different energy when using. He will be age 2 in January, but has been brushing since age 12 weeks, so no problem. His teeth are amazing —of course, zero sugar and carbs, just raw with some vegetation and herbs. I will order a Shungite toothbrush for myself."

Real-Time Analysis Results

Every single test we've conducted with professional equipment shows INSTANT results - not overnight or 3 days:
- Chlorine nullification: Immediate
- Fluoride neutralisation: Immediate
- Balancing pH for your unique body/diet
- Balancing alkalinity and pH for your unique body/diet
- Bacterial reduction: Studies show a 10-900 times reduction within 30 minutes
- Surface tension lowering for greater hydration: Instant

The Convenience Truth

This instant action is why Shungite is so practical for daily life. You don't need to plan ahead or wait—just add your stones to water and drink immediately for purified, energised, healing water whenever you need it. If you don't like the stones knocking about the bottom of containers, simply slip the Oraphim Toggle on and sip quietly! Although you'll want to share this revolutionary Shungite solution far and wide, not so quietly!

Myth 3: You Need 100 Grams Per Litre

We've met people who tried Shungite and gave up, saying it 'didn't work.' When asked about their ratios, they were simply using so much it created a purging effect. A little Shungite goes a long way.

Our Experiments Revealed:
- pH and Alkalinity: 1 stone showed minimal change. Adding just 2 more stones (3 total) transformed the water immediately
- Chlorine/Fluoride: Only 5 grams of Shungite stones are needed to completely neutralise these contaminants
- Real Requirement: 3-5 gram stones X3 per litre—not 100!

The Truth: More isn't better. A small amount works perfectly. Buy a modest bag and you'll have enough to share with family and friends.

Myth 4: Heavy Metal Leaching Concerns

"Shungite leaches dangerous heavy metals into your water"

I know some of you might be worried about heavy metals

or other concerns you've heard about Shungite. Let me put your mind at ease with the words of Anna Kuzminchuk, who beautifully explains:

"There is a wide range of heavy metals in this table (Shungite composition). Most of these substances are in insoluble form and will not be released into the water, and the concentrations of others are so low that they will not cause harm."

The Fear-Based Misunderstanding

This myth breaks my heart because it's based on a complete misunderstanding of how Shungite actually works, and it's preventing people from experiencing its healing benefits due to misunderstood scientific findings.

Bio-Resonance Quantum Remineralisation vs. Physical Leaching

Here's the crucial distinction that changes everything: Shungite doesn't physically leach minerals into water like a tea bag releasing tea. Instead, it performs what I call "bio-resonance quantum remineralisation"—accessing mineral frequencies from the quantum field and delivering exactly what each person's body needs. This isn't just theory—cutting-edge bio-resonance machines can detect and measure these frequency signatures, showing how Shungite actively balances mineral frequencies in real time based on individual requirements.

The Intelligent Scanning System

Think of Shungite as having the most sophisticated scanning system in the universe. The fullerene energy, spinning billions of times per second, can literally read your cellular mineral deficiencies like an advanced Bio-resonance machine costing thousands of pounds, and access the correct frequencies to restore the body to healthy balance, and this effect can be sustained for a few weeks. This explains why studies documenting 'mineral leaching' showed it mysteriously stopping after two weeks: Shungite wasn't randomly releasing minerals, it was completing its personalised healing programme.

Russian researchers Ulyanova Irina Ilyinichna and Aurika Lukovkina discovered that Shungite can selectively isolate mineral deficiencies in individuals and restore mineral balance through ion exchange. This is personalised medicine at the quantum level!

The Two-Week Study Mystery Solved

Several studies reported elevated mineral levels in the first two weeks of using Shungite, which then dropped suddenly. Researchers couldn't explain this, but now we understand: Shungite was responding to the scientists' own mineral deficiencies. Once their bodies were balanced, the frequencies that delivered the elevated readings stopped.

This isn't leaching—it's healing!

Addressing the Fears

The fear-mongering around Shungite's safety simply isn't supported by the science or by the thousands of people who use it daily with nothing but positive results. But an all-too-quick glance can make us cautious about this carbon, but now you know more than the viral vlogs.

The Beautiful Ion Exchange

Shungite performs what I call "divine ion exchange": your essential minerals stay safely where they belong in your cells, while harmful heavy metals, spent toxins, and free radicals get safely escorted out through your urine in those perfectly sized fullerene "cages."

Safety Studies That Prove the Point

Every legitimate safety study shows that Shungite is completely non-toxic, and Shungite comes with a certificate of safety that states:
- Applications not restricted
- Shungite Rock-non-toxic
- Ecologically Safe
- No special requirements for methods of transport

In fact, it's lipophilic, able to go where other antioxidants cannot, and unlike other antioxidants, which can cause harm at high doses, Shungite remains completely safe even at concentrations 10,000 times higher than normal.

You literally cannot overdose on Shungite's healing power!

The Beneficial Minerals Truth

When studies show 'elevated' minerals like copper, nickel, or arsenic, they fail to mention that these are actually beneficial nutrients your body needs in proper amounts:
- Copper: Essential for immune function, kills bacteria and viruses on contact
- Nickel: A vital micronutrient involved in lipid metabolism and hormonal activity
- Arsenic: Used in traditional medicine for centuries for psoriasis, joint pain, and circulation

The key is that Shungite delivers these in bioavailable, beneficial quantum-frequency forms and quantities, not in harmful chemical forms.

Independent Verification

Our own independent study showed that lead levels did not alter with the Shungite stones we provided for testing. The mineral activity people measure is quantum frequency interaction, its not physical contamination, elevated levels are due to the person conducting the tests needing those specific mineral frequencies.

At Oraphim, we made a startling discovery. Several team members tested water using identical Shungite stones and the same water source. The results? Different for each person. The only variable was the testers themselves. This revolutionary finding confirms that Shungite responds to each individual uniquely—simple stone meets complex human consciousness, creating a personalised interaction. It's a divine partnership designed for your specific needs.

Trust Your Body's Wisdom

If you're still concerned, use the toggle method—no physical contact with water at all, just quantum field interaction.

Myth 5: You Must Replace Your Shungite Regularly

This myth creates repeat customers—great for business, terrible for truth. Here's the reality: Shungite never needs replacing and will continuously nullify harmful chlorine and fluoride in your water.

Why? Shungite isn't like other carbons that absorb and get saturated with toxins. Instead, each piece acts as a portal for fullerene energy. It transforms rather than absorbs, meaning it never becomes 'full' or ineffective.

Consider this: Shungite has been purifying water in Karelia for millions of years without human intervention. No cleaning, no replacing—just continuous transformation.

Many report a deeper connection with Shungite. The Sami tribes received messages from these stones, and I've experienced this communication myself. During quiet moments of gratitude, see what Shungite might share with you about your soul's mission.

Myth 6: Cleaning Crystals And Cleaning Shungite

Crystal sellers often claim that Shungite requires energetic cleansing, but this reveals a fundamental misunderstanding. Unlike crystals, which absorb far-infrared radiation within their lattice, Shungite actually emits far-infrared radiation. It doesn't absorb energy, so it never becomes 'full' or requires cleansing.

This energy emission is visible to a few people. When holding Shungite stones in both hands, they can describe a white energy connecting between the stones—a fascinating demonstration of its active energy.

Scientific studies confirm that Shungite emits more far-infrared radiation than elvan, germanium, or jade (commonly used in saunas). This healing radiation penetrates deep into the skin, preventing ageing and improving various conditions, including acne and freckles.

Perhaps most remarkably, Shungite was used to help traumatised children after the Beslan massacre. Research proved its effectiveness for psychological healing. Russia already uses Shungite in healing rooms for patients—it's time we followed their lead.

Myth 7: Physical Contact Required

"Water has to be in contact with the Shungite to be affected by it"

The Quantum Truth That Changes Everything

This might be the most mind-bending myth of all, and I'm absolutely delighted to shatter it for you! The idea that Shungite needs to physically touch water to transform it is like saying you need to touch the sun to feel its warmth. Ridiculous, right?

Understanding the Invisible Network

Here's what's really happening: we're all living within an invisible medium called the aether—the same field that transmits electromagnetic "waves" everywhere. When you splash your arms in a swimming pool, you create ripples on the water's surface, but you didn't add anything new to the water—you simply disturbed or "perturbed" it.

That's exactly what Shungite does, but at quantum speeds! Those fullerenes spinning at 20-30 billion times per second are creating aether perturbations that transform water, whether Shungite is touching it or placed on the outside of the container or pipe work. Yes, it simply works through the sides of the pipes, bottles, or containers.

Our Game-Changing Toggle Experiments

Let me share our breakthrough discovery that left even

us speechless. Customers began reporting something unexpected to both Oraphim and Nancy at Cosmic Reality: silver-activated Shungite was transforming their water—even without direct contact. The water became bubblier, tasted better, and lost its chlorine smell.

This inspired us to create 'toggles'—hand bands that attach Shungite around taps and water bottles. The results were so impressive that we had to test them scientifically.

Using our Palintest Photometer 7500 (high-end water analysis equipment that counts molecules and even their broken bonds, a big step beyond a simple TDS meter or litmus paper), we designed an experiment to eliminate any possibility of physical contact/contamination. We placed our Oraphim toggles and Shungite stickers on the outside of test tubes—no physical contact with water whatsoever, and only for a second.

The results? Absolutely stunning!

The tap water in our control samples turned yellow when tested (indicating chlorine), but every single Shungite sample remained crystal clear for 5 full days, whether the Shungite touched the water or not. Five days of purified water from quantum field interaction, along with no contact whatsoever!

Real-World Evidence

Oraphim customers have experienced purified water using these methods for years, some defining cancer prognosis, reversing uncurable conditions, becoming physically stronger, gaining greater movement, being energised beyond belief, the testimonials are too many to report, often too amazing to believe, yet every word of them is

true:
- Magan Tyson reported that placing one Oraphim sticker on her cold-water pipe eliminated the chlorine smell and created softer water throughout her entire flat
- Tina found that her toggle on the shower head changed how often she needed to clean scale deposits—from every two weeks to not at all in three months
- Tony reported his boiler temperature rose by 12 degrees just from adding a toggle to his tap
- Rebecca's throat infection cleared up overnight
- Children enjoy drinking water
- Without the toggle, Jo's showers are full of chlorine gas
- Alison's hair is softer, and she has colour returning
- A lady reported remarkably colder water coming from the cold tap
- Jo's mum has long outlived the doctor's rectal cancer prognosis
- Albert's lower blood pressure
- Pamela's mum's new liking for drinking water, and no longer needs antihistamine tablets

The Beautiful Confirmation

Here's the part that gave me goosebumps: after five days, the clear Shungite samples began to yellow, and ten days later, they matched the original tap water sample. The chlorine had been there all along, but Shungite's quantum energy had broken the chemical bonds instantly. As the energy dissipated, the bonds reformed.

This proved beyond any doubt that Shungite works through quantum field effects, not just physical contact! But trying to tape Shungite stones to taps and showerheads isn't easy, so we pioneered the Oraphim Shungite Toggles!

Myth 8: Lack Of Scientific Studies

"There are no real scientific studies supporting Shungite's benefits"

The Overwhelming Evidence Mountain

This might be the most easily dispelled myth of all because the scientific evidence for Shungite and the effectiveness of fullerenes is absolutely overwhelming! The problem isn't a lack of studies—it's that people don't know where to look for them or how to interpret them. Shungite, being a completely unique stone, contains a Nobel Prize-winning molecule that's called a fullerene. These are very rare molecules to be found here on Earth, but Shungite is the link, as it is naturally found only in the Shungite region of Karelia, where science meets nature and studies go deeper.

Russian Academy of Sciences Treasure Trove

Let's start with the obvious: The Russian Academy of Sciences has been studying Shungite for decades, with remarkable publications including:
- Professor Inostrantsev's groundbreaking work from 1877-1886
- V. Sokolov and Y. Kalinin's comprehensive studies from 1956-1990
- Professor G. V. Andrievsky Institute of Physiologically Active Compounds research in Medicinal Chemistry, Nanobiochemistry and Nanotechnology applications for Shungite-derived fullerenes
- Dr Nina Kolesnikova, head of cardiology (inc diabetes, hypertension and infectious diseases) at Moscow-based sanatorium

- Countless medical and geological studies from Karelia institutions

Visit Oraphim's website (www.oraphimshungite.com) for an extensive collection of Shungite studies—we continuously update it with the latest research findings.

The Nobel Prize Foundation

Fullerenes won the Nobel Prize in Chemistry in 1996! The foundational research was so groundbreaking that Robert F. Curl, Harold W. Kroto, and Richard E. Smalley received science's highest honour.

International Research Explosion

Rice University and Kazan Federal University (2016): Developed Shungite-based compounds capable of extracting radioactive caesium and strontium from water —crucial for Fukushima cleanup efforts.

National Institute of Health (Multiple studies): Published research showing fullerenes have:
- Anti-inflammatory properties
- Antiviral capabilities
- Antioxidant power exceeding anything previously known
- Anti-HIV properties
- Heart inflammation treatment potential
- Anti-bacterial
- Anti-inflammatory
- Detox properties
- Snake venom antidote (In ancient days is was known as "Viper Stones")
- Vaccine and medical toxicity nullification

The Medical Evidence Avalanche

PubMed Study (February 2023): Seda Beyaz's team demonstrated that C60 fullerene nanoparticles are effective for treating heart inflammation, concluding they are a "promising and potentially effective therapy for heart diseases."

Belgorod Region Sanatorium Study: 154 COPD patients showed remarkable improvement using Shungite solutions, with many reducing or eliminating medication dependency. Try this remarkable steam therapy at home: Add Shungite to boiling water, cover your head with a towel, and inhale the steam over the bowl. This provides rapid respiratory relief and helps reduce cold and flu symptoms.

Military Medical Academy Study: Professor A. Sosyukin documented increased immune function in over 500 patients, including those with acute poisoning from the Chernobyl accident.

The Water Purification Research

Moscow State University Studies (Oleg Mosin): Documented specific removal rates for dozens of contaminants, with results like:
- Iron: 95% removal
- Lead: 85% removal
- Radioactive strontium: 97% removal
- Dioxins: 97% removal

Journal of Water Chemistry and Technology (October 2020): L.A. Deremeshko's team published substantial studies demonstrating Shungite's disinfecting effects and fluoride-removal capabilities.

The Electromagnetic Research

Rainer Schneiders' NIH Study: Used double-blind methodology to prove Shungite dramatically reduces the harmful effects of mobile phones on heart rate variability, cortisol levels, and blood oxygenation.

Dancook University, Korea: Confirmed fullerenes' ability to absorb microwave irradiation, protecting nervous systems from EMF damage. You are a body of water, absorbing all these harmful waves.

EMF protection is explored fully in the companion book 'EMF: Poisoned to Harmonised'.

The Longevity Studies

2012 Rat Studies: C60 fullerenes - naturally found in Shungite - extended life by 90%—the most dramatic longevity increase ever recorded in scientific literature. Oraphim's muscle testing revealed that silver-activated Shungite outperformed all alternatives—including silver-infused synthetic C60 fullerenes. Nature always wins over laboratory versions!

Multiple Cancer Studies: Research from 1998-2007 showed fullerenes inhibit HIV replication and kill cancer cells without harming healthy tissue.

The Academic Avalanche

A simple search for "fullerenes" plus any medical condition yields numerous peer-reviewed studies. The evidence isn't lacking—it's abundant, growing, and consistently positive.

The Living Laboratory

Beyond formal studies, we have thousands of testimonials from real people experiencing real results:

- Thyroid conditions reversing after decades
- Respiratory issues clearing in days, including reversing both COPD and cancer
- Chronic pain disappearing overnight
- Energy levels soaring
- Sleep quality dramatically improving
- Lower blood pressure
- Outliving cancer prognosis

The Suppression Reality

The real question isn't whether studies exist—it's why this information isn't more widely known. When natural solutions threaten pharmaceutical profits, information gets suppressed, discredited, or ignored.

But truth has a way of surfacing, and Shungite's truth is becoming impossible to ignore.

Your Personal Research Project

As you begin working with Shungite, remember that you're joining a global research project spanning centuries. From ancient Karelian healers to modern Nobel Prize winners, from Russian Tsars to everyday people seeking better health—you're part of an unbroken chain of discovery.

Document your experiences, trust your results, and add your voice to the growing chorus of evidence that Shungite is exactly what our world needs right now.

The Truth Sets You Free

These myths and misunderstandings have been holding people back from experiencing Shungite's full potential for far too long. Now that you know the truth, you're free to explore, experiment, and experience the remarkable benefits that await you.

Remember: Shungite works instantly, whether it touches water or not, in any grade you choose, without harmful side effects, and with overwhelming scientific support. Everything else is just noise that keeps you from discovering your own miraculous transformation.

Trust the science, trust your experience, and most importantly, trust that you've been guided to this knowledge for a reason. Your journey with Shungite is just beginning, and the best is yet to come!

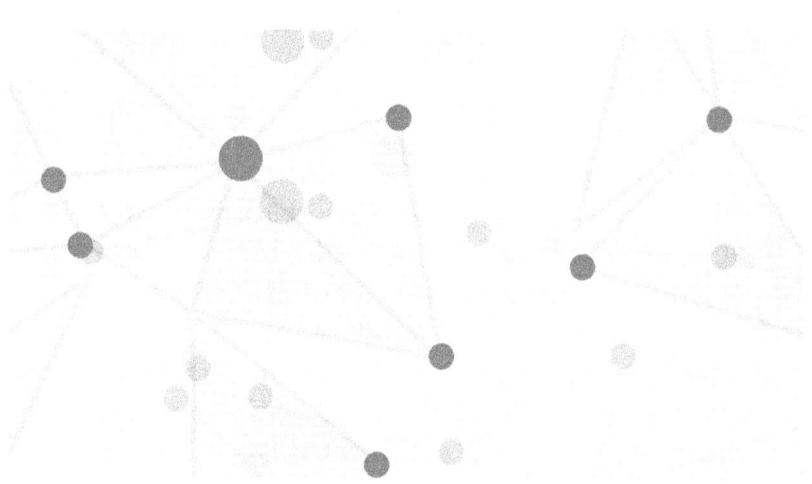

CHAPTER 5: WATER PURIFICATION MECHANISMS

"This water cures various cruel illnesses, in particular: scurvy, morbid depression, gall, stomach weakness, vomiting, diarrhoea, stones, kidneys, and has great power against other illnesses."
— Peter the Great, 1719

I sn't it absolutely wonderful that over 300 years ago, a Russian Tsar recognised what we're only now beginning to understand scientifically? Peter the Great didn't need peer-reviewed studies to see that Shungite water was performing miracles—he could witness the transformations with his own eyes, just as you're about to understand the elegant mechanisms behind these "impossible" healings.

My dear explorer, prepare to have your mind completely blown by the sophisticated intelligence operating within every single piece of Shungite. What you're about to discover will forever change how you think about water, healing, and the quantum magic happening right in your hands.

Chemical Bond Breaking At The Molecular Level

The Quantum Sledgehammer of Healing

Forget everything you thought you knew about water purification! Most filters try to trap or absorb toxins like a net catching fish, but Shungite? Oh, Shungite is far more elegant, intelligent and powerful—it literally breaks the molecular bonds of harmful chemicals, rendering them completely harmless.

The 20-Billion-Times-Per-Second Miracle

Picture this: those magnificent fullerenes spinning at

20-30 billion revolutions per second are like the most sophisticated molecular hammers in the universe, shattering the chemical bonds that hold toxic compounds together. It's not filtration—it's transformation at the atomic level!

When our fullerenes encounter a chlorine molecule, they don't politely ask it to leave or try to trap it in a corner. No! They break its bonds so completely that the chlorine simply ceases to exist as a harmful entity. It's quantum demolition and reconstruction all in one beautiful process.

The Proof That Made Us Giddy!

Remember our famous test tube experiment? We placed Shungite toggles and stickers on the outside of test tubes—no physical contact whatsoever—and watched as the water remained crystal clear for 5 full days, while our control samples turned yellow from chemical contamination.

But here's the part that gave me absolute goosebumps: after five days, the clear samples began to yellow again, and by day ten, they matched the original contaminated water perfectly. The chemicals had been there all along, but Shungite's quantum energy had broken their bonds so completely that they couldn't cause harm. While it passes through your body, or it is used to wash over you each day.

As the energy field dissipated, the bonds slowly reformed. This wasn't absorption or filtration—this was molecular bond manipulation at the quantum level!

The Speed of Quantum Healing

While conventional water treatments work slowly over hours or days, Shungite's bond-breaking happens faster than you can blink. Quicker than the time it takes to make a cup of tea, and it continues for a while as the harmful left spinning molecular structures are dismantled for a full five days. That's not just purification—that's quantum alchemy!

This is why animals trust Shungite water over tap water every time! And they can tell!

Why This Changes Everything

Traditional filters quickly saturate and stop working, but Shungite's bond-breaking mechanism never reaches "full" because it's not storing anything—it's transforming everything. The toxins don't pile up somewhere waiting to be discarded; they're literally changed into harmless components that your body can safely process or eliminate.

This is why Shungite never needs to be replaced. Ever. The mechanism that worked billions of years ago is still working today, and it will work for billions more years. Talk about sustainable technology!

Surface Tension Reduction And Hydration Enhancement

The Secret to True Hydration

Here's something that will revolutionise your understanding of hydration: it's not about how much water you drink—it's about how well your cells can actually absorb it. And this, my soon-to-be-hydrated reader, is where Shungite performs one of its most beautiful miracles.

The Surface Tension Revolution

Dr Patrick Flanagan, an inventor with over 300 patents, made a remarkable discovery: all remote civilisations known for exceptional longevity shared one common factor in their drinking water—lowered surface tension. This isn't a coincidence; this is the key to cellular hydration!

Shungite instantly lowers water's surface tension, and I mean instantly. The moment those spinning fullerenes interact with H_2O molecules, the water becomes eager to penetrate your cells instead of just flowing past them like a stranger.

The Hydration Paradox Solved

Have you ever wondered why you can drink the "recommended" two litres of water per day and still feel chronically dehydrated? It's because most people are flooding their systems with poor-quality water that their cells simply can't absorb!

As Dr R. Cywes explains, this creates a heartbreaking situation where people are literally losing their life-saving electrolytes while remaining dehydrated at the cellular level. To me, it's a bit cult-like to have such an unattainable goal of 2 litres a day. But Shungite water? Your cells recognise it like a long-lost friend and welcome it home, it does its job, and you don't need to pee all the time.

The Quality Over Quantity Truth

Shungite water converts notice something remarkable: they drink less but look and feel better hydrated. This isn't a coincidence—it's science.

Shungite lowers water's surface tension, allowing superior cellular absorption. Instead of forcing down litres that pass straight through, you achieve complete hydration with smaller amounts. Think gentle rain soaking into soil versus a fire hose creating runoff. Less water, better results. This efficient hydration delivers a youthful complexion and transforms ordinary water into a life-giving elixir.

The Cellular Welcome Mat

When surface tension is properly lowered, several magical things happen simultaneously:
- Better nutrient uptake: Your cells can finally absorb the minerals they've been craving
- Effective waste removal: Toxins get escorted out instead of lingering around
- Enhanced energy: Properly hydrated cells function like well-oiled machines
- Improved skin: That healthy glow comes from the inside out
- Energise cells: Complete healthy life cycles, including apoptosis (programme cell death), anti-cancer

The EZ and Far-Infrared Water Connection

Dr Gerald Pollack's revolutionary research reveals how water transforms under far-infrared light. His team discovered that this exposure creates 'liquid crystal water'—a structured form with superior detoxifying properties.

Shungite appears to create this special fourth phase of water (H_3O_2) through its natural emission of far-infrared frequencies. This isn't just hydration—it's cellular energy production and molecular-level detoxification.

Your body can extract energy from this structured water, just as plants harness energy through photosynthesis. Think of it as drinking liquid sunshine—that's what Shungite water offers your cells.

What's Next: Vitamin C Purification and the Key to Youthful Skin

Is there no end to Shungite's water-transforming powers? Here's another way it makes you look younger and feel better.

While expensive serums tout Vitamin C as the latest anti-ageing breakthrough, Shungite offers something better. Its fullerenes are 172 times more powerful than Vitamin C as antioxidants. Users report visibly younger-looking, tighter skin—without the hefty price tag.

Ditch the expensive serums. Save money. Look great. Just another reason why Shungite belongs in your home.

The Taste Test Proof

Here's something beautiful you can experience immediately: Shungite water tastes noticeably different—softer, smoother, more satisfying. Children and animals instinctively prefer it because their bodies recognise its superior quality.

Taste tests were conducted across sixty miles of different regional waters, and every single sample instantly improved dramatically with Shungite treatment. The difference isn't subtle—it's obvious and delightful, and on the same day when everyone got together just for an evening.

Bacterial And Viral Elimination Processes

The Microscopic Battlefield Victory

Now we're entering truly fascinating territory! Shungite doesn't just clean water—it wages war against harmful microorganisms with the precision of a quantum-guided missile system and the gentleness of a loving mother protecting her children.

The 30-Minute Miracle

Studies show that within just 30 minutes of Shungite contact, the concentration of Group D Streptococcus decreases by 10-100 times, and Group A Streptococcus (the nasty ones causing scarlet fever and rheumatism) plummet by an astounding 900 times! But remember that Shungite works instantly, while the scientists capturing the data are experiencing lag in their testing methods.

Think about that: in the time it takes to watch a TV programme, Shungite has identified, isolated, and neutralised dangerous bacteria that could cause serious illness. This isn't just water purification—it's biological protection at the highest level. This was experienced when the lady drank from her bottle with the Oraphim Toggle around it, and her throat was better after months of infection.

The Biofilm Breakthrough

Here's something that will amaze pet owners: add three tiny Shungite stones to your cat's water bowl, and that slimy bacterial biofilm that usually forms on top simply doesn't appear. Ever. Your pets are getting cleaner, safer water without any effort on your part.

But how does this work? The mystery is beautiful and profound.

The Depolarisation Theory

Some researchers suggest that fullerenes trap bacteria

in their cage-like structures and then depolarise them, rendering them completely harmless. But here's the puzzling part: the bacteria are much larger than the fullerenes, so this physical trapping shouldn't be possible.

This suggests something far more sophisticated is happening—a quantum-level interaction that we're only beginning to understand. The fullerenes might be affecting the bacteria's electromagnetic signature, essentially "disconnecting" their harmful properties without physical contact.

The Antiviral Arsenal

Research has shown that fullerenes possess remarkable antiviral properties. Germ Terrain theory gets Shungite responding appropriately:
- HIV inhibition: Studies from 1998 showed fullerenes prevent HIV replication
- Multiple viral strains: The antiviral action isn't limited to one type of virus
- Cellular protection: Healthy cells remain unharmed while viral activity is stopped

The Immune System Partnership

But perhaps most beautifully, Shungite doesn't just kill harmful microorganisms—it supports your body's natural immune function. Professor A. Sosyukin's study of over 500 patients showed increased immune function, including those recovering from acute radiation poisoning.

This isn't chemical warfare against your body's natural flora; it's intelligent support for your immune system's own protective mechanisms.

The Living Water Ecosystem

What emerges is water that doesn't just lack harmful organisms—it actively supports beneficial biological processes. Animals thrive on Shungite water, with reports of:
- Enhanced reproduction: Fish in Shungite-treated tanks reproduce more successfully
- Improved growth: Livestock and fish show better health and development
- Increased vitality: Pets display more energy and better coat quality, and calmer temperament

The Agricultural Miracle

When used with plants and crops:
- Faster germination: Seeds sprout more quickly in Shungite water
- Higher % of germination (100% in Oraphim Study)
- Healthier growth: Plants show increased vigour and disease resistance
- Higher yields: Potato crops increased significantly in controlled studies
- Better quality: Vegetables grow larger and more nutritious

This isn't just water—it's life-enhancing liquid that supports biological flourishing at every level.

Heavy Metal And Toxin Removal Pathways

The Molecular Cleanup Crew

Now we reach perhaps the most crucial mechanism of all, especially in our toxin-saturated modern world. Shungite's approach to heavy metals and toxins is so elegant, so intelligent, that it makes conventional detoxification methods look primitive by comparison.

The Intelligent Ion Exchange

Forget harsh chelation therapies that strip everything from your body indiscriminately or distilled water that's "magnetically" clearing your cells of all their beneficial minerals, as exposed by Dr Mercola's 300-patient study. Shungite performs what I call "divine ion exchange"—it somehow knows exactly which minerals you need to keep and which toxic elements you need to get rid of.

Your essential minerals stay safely in your cells, where they belong, while harmful heavy metals such as lead and other toxins are gently escorted out through your urine in perfectly sized fullerene "cages." It's like having the most sophisticated, loving security system for your body.

Recycling the Free Radicals

Every other detox protocol simply eliminates free radicals —waste removal, nothing more. Shungite fullerenes take a revolutionary approach: molecular rehabilitation.

Here's how they save the day: Fullerenes attract free radicals, then intelligently donate or remove electrons based on each molecule's needs. The result? Former free radicals become useful again for your body. It's cellular recycling at its finest.

The 30-Times-More-Powerful Truth

Professor Andrievsky's research revealed that Shungite is 30 times more effective than activated charcoal at recycling/removing free radicals and antioxidants safely from the body. But unlike charcoal, which works through simple absorption, Shungite transforms toxins at the quantum level.

The Quantum Scanning System

Those fullerenes, spinning billions of times per second, act like quantum scanners, reading your cellular composition and identifying exactly what needs to be removed, and what needs to be preserved or supplemented. This isn't random—it's intelligent, personalised healing at the molecular level.

Russian researchers discovered that Shungite can "selectively isolate mineral deficiencies in individuals and restore mineral balance through ion exchange." Think about the implications: personalised medicine delivered by a rock that's supposedly billions of years old!

The Fullerene Onion Effect

Djuro Koruga's 1997 patent revealed that fullerenes can be layered up to 70 times inside themselves like Russian nesting dolls, creating multiple protective shells around radioactive particles. This "fullerene onion" can trap radiation and create what he calls "radiation absorbing storage molecules."

Imagine: nature created the perfect containment system for our most dangerous pollutants billions of years before we needed it!

What's remarkable to add here is that the radioactive particles are the smallest particles in existence, and Shungite gets more powerful the smaller it gets - so it's not about having big chunks, as the tiniest pinch of powder packs a powerful punch!

The Safe Elimination Pathway

Here's the beautiful part: the fullerenes are the perfect size to pass through your kidneys and be safely eliminated in your urine. Studies show that polyhydroxy fullerene molecules have a size of 1.3 nanometers—small enough to pass through your system without causing any blockages or complications.

The toxins get packaged into tiny molecular suitcases and gently escorted out. No drama, no harsh side effects—just smooth, efficient removal. Your detox protocol becomes so simple, you've probably already started without realising it.

The Lipophilic Advantage

Unlike many detoxification agents that can only work in water-based environments, Shungite is lipophilic—it can reach where other antioxidants cannot, including fatty tissues where many toxins hide. This means comprehensive detoxification at every level of your biology.

The Overdose-Proof Safety

Perhaps most remarkably, studies show that even at concentrations 10,000 times higher than normal doses, Shungite causes absolutely no negative effects on cells. You literally cannot overdose on its healing power!

This gives you the freedom to use Shungite without worry. It will do its best for you and give your body exactly what it needs for detoxification and repair—all at once, without delay.

The Quantum Intelligence

What emerges from all this research is a picture of Shungite as a quantum intelligence system that somehow knows:
- Which toxins to remove and which minerals to preserve
- How much of each beneficial element your body needs
- When to work aggressively and when to work gently
- How to customise its effects for each individual person

This isn't random chemistry—it's conscious, caring, intelligent healing.

Your Personal Transformation System

As you begin working with Shungite water, remember that you're not just drinking purified H_2O. You're inviting a quantum intelligence system into partnership with your body's own healing mechanisms.

Every sip is a conversation between ancient cosmic wisdom and your cellular intelligence. Every glass is an opportunity for transformation, healing, and renewal at the deepest possible level.

The mechanisms we've explored—chemical bond breaking, surface tension reduction, bacterial elimination, free radical recycling and toxin removal—all work together in perfect harmony to create something that transcends simple water purification.

You're not just cleaning your water; you're elevating it to its highest potential and, in doing so, elevating your own biological systems to function as they were divinely designed to function.

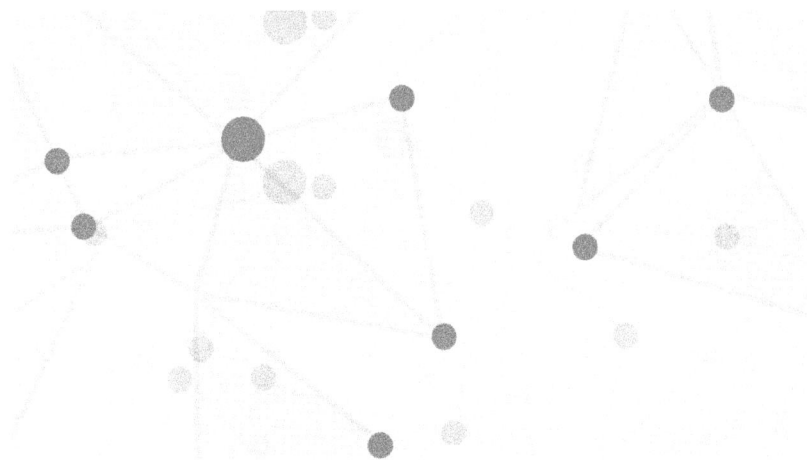

CHAPTER 6: PRACTICAL APPLICATIONS AND METHODS

"Simply use a few stones to activate the water (minimum 3 per container), which can be left for a maximum tasting experience of three days to infuse with healing fullerenes, but you can drink it straight away and it will still be highly effective, purified and healing."

Oh my dear water lover, this is where the magic truly begins! You've learned the science and understand the mechanisms; now it's time to bring this ancient wisdom into your modern life. What I'm about to share with you are the practical secrets I've discovered through years of experimentation, testing, and witnessing countless transformations.

These aren't just instructions—they're keys to unlocking a completely new relationship with water that will ripple through every aspect of your health and wellbeing. So grab your favourite cup of tea (preferably made with Shungite water, of course!), and let's dive into the practical magic together.

Different Forms Of Shungite For Water Treatment

The Beautiful Variety of Options

One of the most wonderful things about Shungite is that it works its magic in so many different forms. Whether you prefer the traditional approach of stones in your water or the innovative convenience of our water transformation toggles, there's a method that's perfect for you.

Raw Stones: The Classic Approach

Black Shungite Chips and Nuggets. These are your workhorses—affordable, effective, and absolutely reliable. Don't let anyone convince you that these humble black stones are somehow "lesser." Some of our most remarkable healing stories come from people using simple black Shungite chips!

- Perfect for: Daily drinking water, large containers, family usage
- Quantity needed: Just three small stones are often enough (remember, Shungite is social and works better in groups!)
- Cost advantage: Maximum benefit for your budget
- Longevity: Literally forever—these stones will outlast you and your grandchildren just as they worked for our ancestors before us.

Elite Shungite Stones. Beautiful, silvery, and undeniably special, Elite stones work only a few seconds faster than their black cousins, and, being quite sharp, it's best not to put them in drink bottles in case of accidental swallowing. If you feel drawn to them, trust that calling—but please don't feel you need them for excellent results. The key is to use at least 3 of each stone.

- Perfect for: bathing, meditation practices
- Investment consideration: Lovely if budget allows, but not essential
- Unique properties: More brittle and sharper, so handle with care

Shungite Powder: The Rapid Response Team

The Dust of Miracles. Even the natural dust that comes off Shungite stones is incredibly powerful. This isn't waste— it's concentrated healing potential!

- Instant action: a pinch of powder works even faster than stones
- Versatile applications: Can be mixed into drinks, foods, or used for steam inhalations

- Tiny amounts needed: A pinch goes a remarkably long way
- Perfect for: Acute situations requiring immediate response

Safety note: A little goes a long way! Start with tiny amounts—your body will guide you to the right dosage.

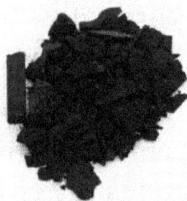

Figure 5: Shungite Dust

Revolutionary Toggles: The Quantum Solution

Our Game-Changing Innovation: These brilliant little devices attach around taps, water bottles, or any container using simple elastic bands. No physical contact needed—pure quantum field interaction!
- Ultimate convenience: No stones to manage or clean if algae growth happens from contact with sunlight
- Quantum proof: Our test tube experiments proved they work without contact
- Travel-friendly: Perfect for bottles, hotel taps, restaurant water
- Family-wide coverage: One on the main tap benefits everyone
- Chlorine gases in showers and bathing are nullified

Toggle testimonials:

*"My boiler temperature rose by 12 degrees
with just a toggle on my tap!"*
*"Haven't had to clean scale from my shower head
in three months since adding the toggle"*
*"The water throughout our entire flat improved
with one sticker on the cold water pipe"*

Silver Activated Shungite Sticker for EMF Protection and Water Activation: The Invisible Protectors

Precision Application Technology Our silver-activated Shungite stickers also work through surfaces, transforming water in pipes, bottles, and containers through quantum field effects.

- Discrete protection: Nobody even knows they're there
- Permanent installation: Stick once, benefit forever
- Pipe applications: Transform your entire water supply at the source
- Professional results: Independent testing confirmed their effectiveness (Dr Klinghardt Method)

Speciality Applications

Bath and Shower Enhancement
- Loose stones in cloth bags: Create a Shungite bath experience
- Shower head attachments: Toggles work beautifully here
- Whole-house applications: Stickers on main water lines

Agricultural and Pet Applications
- Livestock water: Dramatically improves animal health
- Garden irrigation: Plants show remarkable improvement
- Pet bowls: Just a few small stones keep water fresh and healthy

Dosage Guidelines And Safety Protocols

The "Less is More" Principle

Here's something that might surprise you: with Shungite, more isn't necessarily better. This isn't like vitamins, where you might need specific amounts—Shungite is intelligent and gives you exactly what you need.

The Three-Stone Rule

For Daily Drinking Water:
- Minimum effective dose: Just three small stones clustered together
- Maximum recommended: No need to overdo it, buy large amounts for small containers
- The social aspect: Shungite works better in groups—think of it as a "sociable" stone

Why three? Three stones create a coherent quantum field together. One stone on its own would be lonely and energetically less active. It's like the difference between one person singing and a beautiful harmony trio!

Container Size Guidelines

1-2 Litre Containers:
- 3-5 small stones (thumb-size or smaller)
- 1 toggle attachment
- 1 sticker on the outside

Large Family Containers (3-5 litres):
- 5-8 small stones
- Multiple toggles if desired
- Strategic sticker placement

Single Serving (1 cup):
- 3 small stones
- Toggle on the bottle
- Or pre-made Shungite water

Timing Protocols

Immediate Use: Drink right away—it's already effective! Optimal Taste: 3-24 hours for maximum flavour development. Maximum Efficacy

Safety Protocols That Give You Peace of Mind

The Wonderful Truth About Shungite Safety:
- Non-toxic at any reasonable dose: Studies show safety even at 10,000x normal concentrations
- No negative interactions: Works harmoniously with medications and supplements
- Self-regulating: Your body takes what it needs and ignores the rest
- Long-term use: Perfectly safe for daily consumption indefinitely

Preparation Guidelines

First Use Preparation:

1. Gentle rinse: Quick wash under running water to remove any shipping dust
2. No harsh cleaners: Soap and chemicals aren't necessary
3. Trust the process: Shungite is naturally antibacterial and self-cleaning

Ongoing Maintenance:
- Occasional rinse: When you remember, but not essential

- No replacement needed: Ever! These stones will outlast you
- Keep out of sunlight, and give stones and containers a wash if algae forms
- Storage: Anywhere convenient—they're not fragile (except Elite stones)

Special Situation Protocols

For Acute Detox Needs:
- Powder method: Tiny pinch in water or raw honey and use each day for 7 dates, then have a day off
- Listen to your body: It will guide you to the right approach

For Sensitive Individuals:
- Start slowly: Begin with one cup of Shungite water in the morning
- Gradual increase: Add more Shungite water as your body adjusts
- Trust your instincts: If something feels too intense, reduce and adjust
- If you're needing to pee a lot, reduce the amount of water you're drinking

For Travel:
- Toggles are perfect: Work on any bottle or tap
- Small stone collection: Carry a few in a small pouch
- Hotel applications: Toggles on bathroom taps and showers transform the entire experience
- Wear a Shungite bracelet or necklace, which you can tap onto your glass of water for instant effective purification and transformation

Comparative Analysis With Other Filtration

Methods

The Great Water Treatment Showdown

After years of testing, research, and witnessing real-world results, I can honestly say that nothing comes close to Shungite's comprehensive benefits. But let me show you the evidence so you can see for yourself why this ancient solution outperforms everything modern technology has created.

Traditional Carbon Filters: The Disappointing Standard

What They Promise:
- Basic contaminant removal
- Improved taste and odour
- "Cleaner" water

The Reality:
- Basic carbon filters tested are only 10% effective at removing most contaminants
- Expensive replacement cycle: New filters every few months
- Environmental waste: Non-recyclable cartridges pile up in landfills
- No life force: Water remains energetically dead
- Chemical retention: Many toxins pass right through

Our Direct Comparison: We tested a 15-stage filter against Shungite using professional equipment. The results? Even a pinch of common black Shungite outperformed the complex, expensive filter system!

Reverse Osmosis: The Mineral Stripper

What They Promise:
- Removal of virtually all contaminants

- "Pure" water
- Long-term filtration solution

The Devastating Reality:
- Strips all minerals: Including the beneficial ones your body needs
- Creates "hungry" water: Pulls minerals from your cells
- Energetically dead: No life force or beneficial frequencies
- Expensive maintenance: Membrane replacements and system servicing
- Water waste: Produces 3-5 gallons of waste for every gallon of "pure" water
- Still no memory clearing: Past contamination patterns remain

Why This Matters: Your body needs minerals to function. RO water is like giving someone a house, then removing all the furniture—technically "clean," but completely unusable for its intended purpose.

Expensive Electrical Systems: The Chemical Creators

What They Promise:
- "Alkaline" water for better health
- Electrical enhancement
- Scientific-sounding benefits

The Shocking Truth:
- Creates chlorine: As metal plates oxidise, they produce the very chemical you're trying to avoid!
- Thousands of dollars: For systems that actually add toxins to your water
- Ongoing electricity costs: Your water purification increases your electric bill
- Complex maintenance: Professional servicing required
- Marketing over science: Lots of claims, little real benefit

Real User Report: Amanda Bobbett, a former Kangen saleslady, publicly demonstrated how these systems create chlorine in the water. You're literally paying thousands to poison yourself!

UV and Chemical Sterilisation: The Life Killers

What They Promise:
- Bacterial and viral elimination
- "Safe" water
- Chemical disinfection

The Problems:
- Kills everything: Good bacteria along with bad
- Chemical residues: Chlorine, chloramines, and other disinfectants remain
- No toxin removal: Bacteria die, but toxins stay
- Ongoing chemical exposure: You're drinking the sterilizing agents
- Dead water syndrome: All life force eliminated

The Economic Reality

Over 10 Years:
- Traditional filters: £500-1,500 in replacement costs
- Reverse osmosis: £200-500 in membrane replacements plus wasted water costs
- Electrical systems: £3,000-8,000 initial cost plus electricity and maintenance
- Chemical treatments: Ongoing chemical purchase costs
- Shungite: £10 one-time investment. Done. Forever. (current availability, but it's predicted to be more valuable than gold in the future, and you might see why now!)

The Health Comparison

Traditional Methods:
- Remove small % bad things
- Often remove good things too
- Add unwanted chemicals or processes
- Create energetically dead water
- No customisation for individual needs

Shungite Method:
- Removes/neutralises all harmful elements
- Adds beneficial frequencies and energy
- Intelligent ion exchange preserves needed minerals
- Creates living, structured water
- Adapts to each person's unique requirements

The Environmental Victory

Other Methods:
- Produce ongoing waste (filters, membranes, chemicals)
- Require energy consumption
- Need replacement parts and servicing
- Often waste water in the process

Shungite:
- Zero waste production
- No energy requirements
- Nothing ever needs replacing
- Actually improves environmental water quality where used

The Convenience Factor

Other Methods:
- Complex installation requirements
- Ongoing maintenance schedules
- Professional servicing needs

- Multiple components to manage

Shungite:
- Drop stones in water or attach toggles
- No installation, no maintenance, no servicing
- Works immediately and continuously
- So simple a child can use it perfectly

Your Clear Choice

Your Journey to Perfect Water Starts Now

You now have everything you need to transform your relationship with water forever. Whether you choose simple stones, convenient toggles, or innovative stickers, you're stepping into a partnership with quantum intelligence that will serve you for the rest of your life.

Remember: start simple, trust the process, and prepare to be amazed by what this ancient mysterious gift can do for your modern life. The water transformation begins with your very next sip!

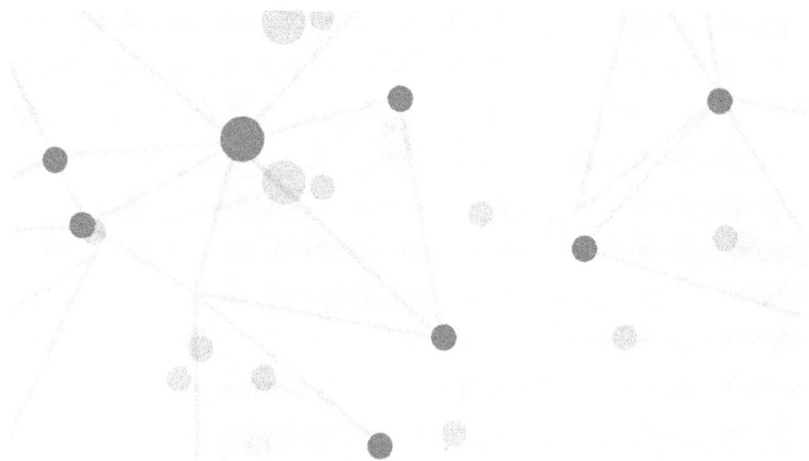

CHAPTER 7:
WATER ANALYSIS
AND TESTING

"The results were visible; the tap water turned yellow because the chlorine that was present reacted with the potassium iodide in the acid solution, which releases the iodine, yet all the Shungite samples remained crystal clear for 5 days, whether the Shungite had physically touched the water or not."

My dear water detective, prepare to become absolutely fascinated by what's actually lurking in your tap water—and utterly amazed by how dramatically Shungite transforms it! What I'm about to share with you are the testing methods and discoveries that left even seasoned scientists speechless.

You see, testing water isn't just about satisfying scientific curiosity (though that's delightfully addictive once you start). It's about witnessing miracles in real-time, proving to yourself that this isn't just a placebo effect or wishful thinking—it's a genuine, measurable, repeatable transformation happening right before your eyes.

So grab your detective hat and let's dive into the wonderful world of water analysis. Trust me, you'll never look at a glass of water or Shungite the same way again!

Laboratory Testing Methodologies

Our Professional-Grade Investigation

When we decided to seriously test Shungite's claims, we didn't mess around with basic test strips (though those have their place, as you'll see). Oh no! We invested in the Palintest Photometer 7500—a high-end water analysis instrument used by laboratories for serious scientific work.

Why did we go to such lengths? Because frankly, the claims about Shungite seemed almost too good to be true, and we needed rock-solid evidence that would convince even the most sceptical scientist. What we discovered exceeded our wildest expectations!

The Game-Changing Experimental Design

Here's where we got really clever. Most people test Shungite by putting stones directly in water, but we suspected something far more extraordinary was happening. So we designed experiments to capture Shungite's quantum effects without the possibility of physical contamination.

The Breakthrough Protocol:
- Shungite soaked water sample (contact time 1 second)
- Sealed test tubes with tap water
- Shungite toggles and stickers attached to the outside of tubes
- Control samples with no Shungite contact
- Professional laboratory analysis over extended time periods

This wasn't just testing—this was quantum detective work!

Chlorine Detection: The Yellow Revelation

The Chemistry Behind the Magic: When chlorine is present in water and you add potassium iodide in an acid solution, it releases iodine, which turns the water yellow. It's a reliable, visual way to detect chlorine, used by professionals for decades.

Our Jaw-Dropping Results:
- Control samples: Turned bright yellow immediately (high chlorine presence)
- All Shungite samples: Remained crystal clear for 5 full days
- No physical contact: Toggles and stickers were on the outside of sealed tubes

- Quantum proof: The effect worked through glass and air!

But here's the part that gave us absolute goosebumps: after 5 days, the clear samples began to yellow, and by day 10, they matched the control samples perfectly. The chlorine had been there all along, but Shungite's quantum field had broken the molecular bonds so completely that they couldn't react chemically.

Additionally, Shungite enhances our body's ability to absorb and utilise the vital iodine we naturally consume in our diet.

Fluoride Testing: The Red Alert System

The Visual Test Protocol: Fluoride testing requires an acid solution with Zirconyl Chloride and Eriochrome Cyanine R, which creates a red colour. When fluoride is present, it degrades this red colour, turning it orange—the more fluoride, the more orange it becomes.

Our Stunning Discovery:
- Contaminated tap water: Turned distinctly orange (fluoride present)
- Shungite-treated water: Remained beautifully red (fluoride neutralised)
- Instant results: Transformation happened immediately
- Consistent pattern: Every Shungite sample showed the same remarkable improvement

pH and Alkalinity: The Personalised Water Phenomenon

Now, here's where we discovered something absolutely extraordinary that will revolutionise how you think about water testing! When most people test pH levels in water, they pop the test strip in, record the answer, and job done—you have your reading. But Shungite alkalinity/pH experimentation isn't straightforward, and what we discovered will blow your mind!

The Experiment That Changed Everything: We conducted controlled experiments using Elite and regular black Shungite, giving different pH readings for different people when using exactly the same stones and the same water source with 15-in-1 test strips.

The Shocking Discovery: Using only one stone each of Elite and black Shungite, we tested twice and got the same reading—but these readings were completely different for each participant! The water was identical, the stones were identical, but the results were uniquely individual.

Then It Got Even More Amazing: When we added extra stones to each cup, the water always made a dramatic difference in both pH/alkalinity. This confirmed that our minimum recommendation of 3 stones is essential for properly transforming the water.

The Mind-Blowing Conclusion: Because the water gives different starting readings using exactly the same stones and water, with the only difference being who is conducting the test, we can scientifically conclude that Shungite really is creating unique water for each person!

Why This Happens: Each of us already has a unique pH/blood group/diet/toxicity profile. When working with a quantum adaptogen such as Shungite, we can create our own quantum pH medical waters, specifically needed to provide a balancing effect for our individual bodies.

What This Means for You:
- Your results will be unique: Don't compare your pH

readings to others
- Trust your body's response: Your individual readings are exactly what you need
- Minimum stone requirement: Always use at least 3 stones together for proper effect
- Personalised medicine: You're receiving customised water therapy at the quantum level

The Scientific Implications: This discovery proves that Shungite isn't just a passive filter—it's an intelligent system that reads your individual biochemistry and creates personalised healing water. This is quantum medicine in action, delivered through a humble black stone!

Multi-Parameter Professional Analysis

What We Measured:
- Hardness levels
- Nitrate content
- Fluoride presence
- Chlorine content
- Alkalinity
- pH stability
- Turbidity (clarity)
- Mineral content changes

The Comprehensive Victory: Shungite outperformed our expensive 15-stage filter in every single category that matters for human health. The filter might have changed some numbers, but Shungite transformed the water's entire biological compatibility profile.

The Consistent Miracle: Every single test confirmed Shungite's remarkable effects. The results weren't just good —they were consistently extraordinary across all variables.

Home Testing Options

Your Kitchen Laboratory

Now, I know not everyone can invest in £10,000 worth of laboratory equipment (though, honestly, after seeing these results, you might be tempted!). The beautiful thing is that many of Shungite's effects are so dramatic that you can witness them with simple, affordable home tests alongside some of the newest water researchers' techniques, such as Veda Austin's simple freezing method.

The 15-in-1 Test Strip Bonanza

Why We Love These: For about £20, you get a comprehensive water testing kit that measures:

1. pH levels
2. Hardness
3. Chlorine
4. Nitrates
5. Nitrites
6. Iron
7. Copper
8. Lead
9. Fluoride
10. And more!
11. Test your tap water as a baseline
12. Add Shungite to one glass, leave another as control
13. Add a cluster of Shungite to another glass
14. Test both after 1, 5, 10, 20 minutes, 2 hours, and 24 hours
15. Document the changes

What You'll Likely See:
- pH optimisation
- Reduction in toxins
- More stable readings over time
- Water trending toward biological compatibility

Veda Austin Freezing Method:

Freeze a water sample of both Shungite and tap water in a clear glass dish for exactly 5 minutes and 20 seconds. Remove and pour away the unfrozen water to reveal a beautiful pattern that will be significantly different from the tap water. What's the water trying to tell you?

The Taste Test: Your Most Sensitive Instrument

Why This Works: Your taste buds are incredibly sophisticated chemical detection devices. Water improvements that instruments might measure in parts per million can be instantly detected by your palate.

The Family Experiment:

1. Blind taste testing: Have family members taste unmarked samples
2. Regional comparison: Test water from different sources
3. Before and after: Same source, with and without Shungite
4. Children's reactions: Kids are especially sensitive to water quality
5. Pet preferences: Animals instinctively choose better water

What You'll Experience:
- Softer, smoother mouthfeel

- Reduced metallic or chemical tastes
- Enhanced refreshment sensation
- Natural preference for Shungite water

The Visual Clarity Test

Simple but Revealing:
- Fill identical clear glasses with treated and untreated water
- Compare visual clarity and any cloudiness
- Look for sediment or floating particles
- Document with photos over time

What Often Happens:
- Shungite water appears clearer and brighter
- Reduced cloudiness and particulates (turbidity)
- More "alive" appearance (hard to describe but easy to see)

The Practical Application Tests

The Flower Power Experiment:
- Cut flowers in Shungite water vs. tap water
- Document longevity and freshness
- Watch how stems stay firmer longer
- Observe reduced bacterial growth in the vase

The Plant Growth Study:
- Water identical plants with different water sources (tap and Shungite water)
- Document growth rates and plant health
- Compare leaf colour and vitality
- Measure time and % of success to germination for seeds

The Pet Preference Test:
- Offer your pets side-by-side water bowls
- Document which they choose consistently

- Observe their overall water consumption
- Note any changes in energy or health

Creative Home Testing Ideas

The Ice Cube Comparison:
- Make ice cubes from treated and untreated water
- Compare clarity, taste, and melting characteristics
- Use in drinks for blind taste comparisons

The Cooking Enhancement Test:
- Cook identical meals with different water sources (especially foods that rehydrate)
- Compare flavour, texture, and cooking times
- Document family preferences and reactions

The Coffee/Tea Transformation:
- Brew identical beverages with different waters
- Compare aroma, flavour, and overall satisfaction
- Often the most dramatic and immediately noticeable difference!

Before And After Comparisons

The Dramatic Transformations We've Witnessed

Nothing prepared us for the sheer magnitude of improvements we'd document. These aren't subtle changes requiring sensitive instruments—these are dramatic, obvious, life-changing transformations that anyone can see, taste, and experience, and there are too many for me to keep up with each week.

Pam Duthie reports a transformation: Her mother, who previously avoided water, now drinks it willingly for the first time in her life. Even better, she hasn't needed

antihistamines throughout spring and summer 2025—
eliminating the health risks from those chemical side
effects entirely.

Long-Term Tracking Results

The Six-Month Studies: Following customers over
extended periods revealed:
- Sustained improvements: Effects don't diminish over
time
- Compounding benefits: Results actually improve with
continued use
- Health improvements: Customers report better hydration
and energy
- Economic benefits: Reduced spending on bottled water
and appliances

The Appliance Longevity Reports:
- Reduced scale buildup: Customers report cleaner
appliances
- Rinse aid in dishwashers is not required
- Extended equipment life: Water heaters and kettles last
longer
- Energy efficiency: Improved heat transfer in water-using
appliances
- Maintenance reduction: Less descaling and repair needed

Shungite's Typical Impact:
- Appliance benefits: Less scale, longer equipment life
- Personal benefits: Softer feeling on skin and hair
- Soap efficiency: Better lathering, less soap needed (more
money savings

Using Shungite in body care products is revolutionary.
Its antibacterial and transformational properties go

beyond surface cleaning—they work at deeper cellular levels. Shungite-infused water penetrates through skin layers, enhancing nutrient absorption (like magnesium in Oraphim Bath Salts) while avoiding harsh chemicals that damage your electromagnetic field—your body's first line of defence.

Fluoride: The Controversial Contaminant

Shungite's Dramatic Effect:
- Typical reduction: 80-95% elimination
- Speed: Instant neutralisation
- Method: Molecular bond breaking, not filtration
- Consistency: Reliable results across all water sources

Health Significance: Artificial fluoride can disrupt vital pineal and thyroid function, affecting brain and body chemistry. Shungite's ability to neutralise it gives your endocrine system a chance to function properly.
- Harmful forms eliminated: Toxic compounds neutralised
- Beneficial forms preserved: Your body gets what it needs
- Intelligent selection: Shungite knows what to keep and what to transform
- No mineral depletion: Unlike RO systems, it doesn't strip everything

The Key Insight: Don't panic if you see mineral readings —ask whether they're beneficial or harmful forms, and remember that Shungite's intelligence transforms toxins while preserving nutrients.

Bacterial Indicators: The Biological Safety Markers

Standard Measurements:
- Coliform bacteria: Indicator of faecal contamination
- E. coli: Specific harmful strain

- Total bacterial count: General microbial load

Shungite's Documented Performance:
- Group A Streptococcus: 900x reduction in 30 minutes
- Group D Streptococcus: 10-100x reduction in 30 minutes
- General bacterial load: Dramatic decreases across all types
- Biofilm prevention: Stops bacterial film formation entirely

What This Means for You: That slimy biofilm in your pet's water bowl disappears, and you're protected from waterborne illnesses that occasionally make it into the drinking water system and could make you seriously ill.

Interpreting Anomalous Results

When Numbers Don't Make Sense: Sometimes test results seem contradictory or unexpected. Here's how to interpret them:

Temporary Mineral Elevation:
- What it looks like: Higher mineral readings in the first 1-2 weeks
- What's really happening: Shungite responding to your body's deficiencies or infections
- When it stabilises: Usually within 2-4 weeks
- Not a problem: This is personalised quantum remineralisation

pH Fluctuations:
- What you might see: pH jumping around initially
- The real story: Shungite optimising for your individual needs
- The end result: More stable, biologically compatible water
- Don't chase numbers: Focus on how the water makes you feel

Individual Variation Between People:
- Why it happens: Each person's biochemistry is unique
- Shungite's response: Adjusts its effects for individual needs
- What to expect: Your results will be different from others using identical stones and water sources
- The bottom line: Trust that your personalised results are exactly what your body needs

The Most Important Test: Your Body's Response

Beyond the Numbers: All the laboratory analysis in the world means nothing compared to how Shungite water makes you feel. Here's what to monitor:

Immediate Effects (First Week):
- Hydration quality: Do you feel more satisfied with less water?
- Energy levels: Any improvement in vitality?
- Skin condition: Softer, more hydrated feeling?
- Digestive comfort: Better stomach response to water?
- Chronic condition improvements: Any ongoing health issues improving?

Medium-Term Changes (2-8 Weeks):
- Sleep quality: Deeper, more restful sleep?
- Mental clarity: Improved focus and thinking?
- Physical comfort: Reduced inflammation or joint stiffness?
- Overall well-being: General sense of improved health?
- Chronic condition improvements: Any ongoing health issues improving?
- Emotional changes: Calmer reactions, more balanced moods, heart-centred feelings?

Long-Term Transformations (2+ Months):
- Chronic condition improvements: Any ongoing health issues improving?
- Energy stability: More consistent energy throughout the day?
- Stress resilience: Better ability to handle daily challenges?
- Intuitive connection: Stronger sense of inner guidance and peace?
- Life direction: Experiencing new opportunities or positive life transformations?

Creating Your Personal Water Quality Journal

Track What Matters:

1. Daily water intake: Quantity and quality of hydration
2. Energy levels: Morning, afternoon, evening ratings
3. Sleep quality: Depth and restfulness scores
4. Physical symptoms: Any changes in ongoing conditions
5. Emotional well-being: Mood, stress levels, overall happiness
6. Intuitive insights: Dreams, meditations, spiritual experiences
7. Personal pH readings: Document your unique patterns over time

Monthly Testing Schedule:
- Week 1: Baseline measurements and initial Shungite introduction
- Week 2: First adaptation period observations and pH personalisation

- Week 4: Stabilisation and optimisation tracking
- Month 3: Long-term transformation documentation
- Month 6: Comprehensive benefit analysis

The Ultimate Test: Trust Your Experience

Your Body Knows: After all the scientific analysis, laboratory testing, and numerical comparisons, the most important indicator is your lived experience. Your body is the most sophisticated testing instrument ever created, capable of detecting improvements that our crude human instruments might miss.

Trust the Process:
- If you feel better: The water is working, regardless of test numbers
- If you're drawn to drink less: Your body recognises superior hydration
- If you're drawn to drink more: Your body recognises superior quality, safe water to drink
- If others notice improvements: The effects are real and noticeable
- If you sleep, think, and feel better: That's the ultimate proof
- If your pH readings are unique: That's exactly what your body ordered

The Scientific and Spiritual Balance: Use testing to satisfy your mind's need for evidence, but trust your body's wisdom to guide your ongoing relationship with Shungite water. Science confirms what ancient wisdom has always known—this remarkable substance is here to help you thrive as the unique, divinely designed body of water that you are.

The discovery that Shungite creates personalised pH and mineral readings for each individual represents a breakthrough in our understanding of quantum medicine. You're not just drinking purified water—you're receiving customised healing frequencies delivered through the most sophisticated natural technology ever discovered.

Your Water Quality Adventure Begins

Armed with this testing knowledge, including the revolutionary understanding of Shungite's personalised pH response, you're now ready to become your own water quality detective! Whether you choose simple home tests or invest in professional analysis, you'll be amazed by the transformations you witness.

Remember: the goal isn't to achieve perfect numbers on a chart—it's to create water that supports your highest health and wellbeing. Let the testing confirm what your body already knows: Shungite water is extraordinary, and your unique results are exactly what you need.

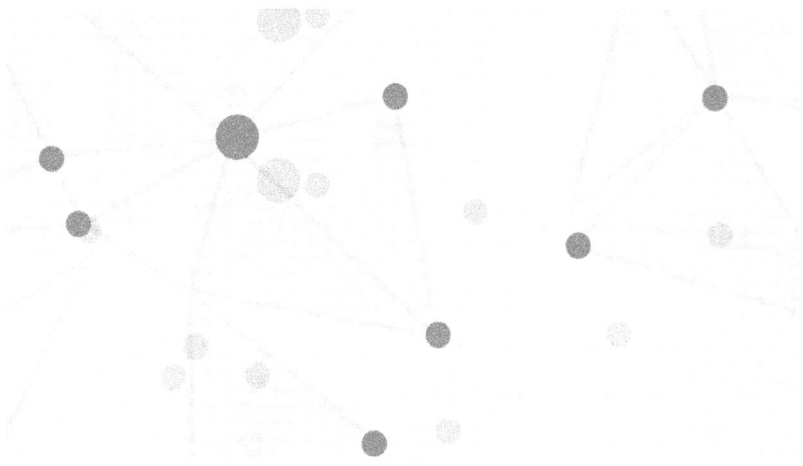

CHAPTER 8:
TESTIMONIALS AND
CASE STUDIES

My beautiful reader, this is where science becomes personal, where laboratory results transform into real human stories, and where hope becomes reality. What you're about to read isn't just data— these are love letters from people whose lives have been fundamentally changed by their relationship with

Shungite water.

Some of these stories will bring tears to your eyes, others will fill you with wonder, and all of them will remind you that miracles aren't just possible—they're happening every single day to ordinary people who dared to trust in something extraordinary.

Prepare to be inspired, amazed, and perhaps most importantly, convinced that your own transformation is not only possible but inevitable.

Compiled User Experiences Extend Beyond Just Water Treatment

The Brain Tumour Miracle That Started It All

Let me begin with the story that changed everything for us—the first profound healing we witnessed, which convinced us that Shungite was far more than just a water purifier.

The Diagnosis: A gentleman we knew was suddenly diagnosed with brain tumours behind both eyes. The doctors gave him three months to live. Can you imagine receiving news like that? The devastation, the fear, the sense of helplessness?

Our Simple Intervention: We gave him black Shungite stones for his drinking water and a laminated patch of Shungite powder to wear in his hat. Nothing fancy, nothing expensive—just humble black Shungite and hope.

The Medical Horror: To everyone's terror, he accidentally received double the prescribed dose of radiation therapy. His family rushed him for emergency liver and kidney function tests, expecting devastating damage.

The Impossible Result: The test results came back completely normal. Not "elevated" or "acceptable"— completely normal. The medical staff was astonished. His family wept with relief.

The Miracle Continues: At the three-month mark, his treatment team said, "Well, whatever you're doing, carry on. We're now giving you a life expectancy of four years due to your improvements and the shrinking of the tumours."

What This Taught Us:
- Black Shungite can achieve miraculous results (this wasn't Elite!)
- Medical treatments become more effective, not less, when combined with Shungite
- The body's resilience increases dramatically
- Hope should never be abandoned, even in the darkest circumstances

The Chronic Fatigue Liberation

Twenty-Four Years of Exhaustion: A woman approached us at an event, sharing that she had suffered from Chronic Fatigue Syndrome for 24 years. Twenty-four years! Can you imagine the frustration, the lost opportunities, the daily struggle just to function?

One Pyramid, One Night: She purchased one of our Oraphim pyramids on Saturday evening and took it home.

Sunday Morning Transformation: She returned to our exhibition stand the very next morning, tears streaming down her face, barely able to speak. Her energy had been completely restored overnight—for the first time in nearly a quarter-century, she woke up feeling truly alive.

The Emotional Impact: Watching this woman's joy was one of the most profound experiences of my life. To witness someone reclaim their vitality after decades of suffering —there simply aren't words adequate to describe that moment of pure, radiant happiness.

The Arthritis Overnight Relief

At a similar event, a gentleman suffering from severe arthritis bought a pyramid for his son. The next morning, he returned amazed—his arthritic pain had eased overnight just from having the pyramid in his home. He immediately purchased one for himself.

The Discovery: The next morning, he returned, amazed to report that his arthritis had eased considerably overnight. Just from being around the pyramid energy field for a few hours, his chronic pain had significantly diminished.

The Ripple Effect. Word spread quickly through the event. People began bringing friends and family to experience the pyramid energy firsthand. We witnessed transformation after transformation that weekend—and now at every event, we help people release pain, clear energy blockages, and restore their natural flow.

For those seeking immediate arthritis relief, there's another option: Oraphim Rescued Balm. This collaboration with Susie works within minutes, consistently surprising first-time users with its rapid effectiveness. Another breakthrough product the world needs to discover.

Water Transformation Stories

Kay's Plant Revelation: *"I've been watering my plants with water with the stones in and all of them are noticeably looking much healthier, including the cactus, and I've not used any plant food."* — Kay, November 2023

The Coffee Shop Miracle: Experiencing the magic of our geodome installations at various events, people consistently commented that the coffee served inside our fullerene-inspired structures was "the best coffee at the event." We later realised that, just by having water inside the fullerene geodome, it was being transformed by the geometric form into something that tasted better!

The Bus Pass Mystery: Maggie carried Shungite powder in her purse and found that her bus pass (with an RFID tracking chip) was affected and wouldn't work until she removed it. The Shungite was providing protection from electromagnetic tracking—something she actually needed for her interdimensional travel practices!

The Well Water Transformation

The Russian Dacha Story: Friends of our Shungite miners bought a rural property but were dismayed to find their well water had a foul hydrogen sulfide smell, high colour, and terrible turbidity.

The Simple Solution: They poured 50 kg of Shungite into the well.

The Remarkable Results:
- Spring transformation: The following spring, the water was crystal clear with no odour
- Three-year timeline: After three years, the water was completely drinkable
- Laboratory confirmation: Pirogov laboratory tests showed only slight iron and manganese elevation—

everything else was perfect
- Bacterial elimination: Complete removal of harmful bacteria and contaminants

The cost-effective off-grid solutions: As more people are moving from urban to rural off-grid communities, these are natural solutions that are a fraction of the cost of conventional water treatment and provide permanent results.

The Thyroid Resurrection

Thirty Years of Medication: Tony from Doncaster had suffered from an underactive thyroid for over three decades, requiring daily Thyroxine medication that only gets stronger over time.

The Simple Solution: He began consistently wearing a silver-activated Oraphim Shungite pendant near his thyroid and drinking from his toggled glass in the evenings.

The Medical Miracle: After three months, his routine thyroid function test showed such improvement that his doctor immediately reduced his Thyroxine prescription by one-third.

Why This Matters: Underactive thyroid is typically considered "incurable" by mainstream medicine and usually only worsens over time. This reversal defied medical expectations and gave this man his life back. Thyroid disruption is often caused by chlorine exposure, and Shungite has been proven to instantly nullify this toxin.

The Lupus Victory

The Progressive Disease: A Lupus patient experienced severe symptoms and required regular HCQ medication to manage her condition. Lupus is an autoimmune disease that typically worsens over time.

Year One with Shungite: After incorporating Shungite into her daily routine, she reduced her HCQ use to just 1 tablet per month.

Year Two Breakthrough: By the second year, she no longer needed any HCQ medication. Her lupus symptoms had completely disappeared.

The Hidden Truth: Research suggests that lupus may be caused by parasites, and Shungite is proven to remove 90% of helminth eggs from the gastrointestinal tract. Did Shungite eliminate the parasite causing her condition? The evidence strongly suggests yes.

The Ganglion Disappearance

Jackie's Quick Fix: *"I got in touch to report my ganglion had dissipated after about four hours in total of a toggle being placed over my ganglion. The last application resulted in a detoxification headache, and then it has now gone. Probably took six applications as the toggle wasn't too comfy on the wrist at that time."*

Four Hours Total: A ganglion that had been troubling her for months disappeared in just four hours of Shungite contact. This wasn't gradual improvement—this was rapid, complete resolution.

The Diabetes Miracle

A man with diabetes recovering from a very recent operation, having had his little toes amputated due to poor blood circulation, was instantly relieved and able to sleep, allowing deep healing.

The Simple Intervention: He received his Shungite package and began using it immediately.

The Healing Acceleration: Within days, he experienced dramatic improvement in sleep and pain relief without opioid medication. When the nurse changed his wound dressings, they were amazed to find his wounds healing unexpectedly quickly.

The Circulation Restoration: Shungite had increased his circulation, allowing blood to flow to his extremities again. His healing accelerated beyond medical expectations.

From Paralysis to Walking

"Jane Osborne was left paralysed from the neck down after a parachute accident. When Shungite stones were placed at her feet, the healing process began. Today, she walks without any aids or support.

Professional Observations

Dr H. Brew's Laboratory Transformation

"When I put my Shungite bracelet on, it transforms my day. I am engaged, inspired, motivated and achieve what I set in motion. My lab work is transformed, with perfect results the first time. How different my day is from what it was before I knew Shungite. I feel I experience my best work on these Shungite-wearing days."

The Professional Impact: Dr Brew, a chemist, noticed that Shungite didn't just affect his personal energy—it transformed his professional performance. Laboratory work became more precise, results more accurate, and his overall effectiveness dramatically improved.

The Consistency Factor: This wasn't a one-time experience. Dr Brew specifically noted that "Shungite wearing days" were consistently his most productive and successful days.

Nurse Caron Barr's Blood Analysis Discovery

The Live Blood Study: Registered Nurse Caron Barr conducted live blood analysis on someone using Nancy Hopkins' S4 (silver-activated Shungite) sticker on their mobile phone.

The Impossible Finding: She discovered a cluster of six stem cells present during the examination. As she explained, "Stem cells are never found in adults—yet there they were."

The Protective Mechanism: When the mobile phone was used, blood cells initially stacked up (normal Wi-Fi damage), but then something remarkable happened: white blood cells immediately arrived to detoxify the damaged cells, and they were released from stacking in super-quick time.

The Professional Conclusion: A medical professional with years of blood analysis experience had never seen anything like Shungite's protective and regenerative effects on human blood.

The Medical Staff Astonishment

The Brain Tumour Case: When our friend with a brain tumour accidentally received double radiation doses, the medical staff was genuinely astonished by his normal liver and kidney function tests.

Professional Expectations: Medical studies show that patients undergoing radiation treatment typically take 2-3 months for liver and kidney function to return to normal levels. With Shungite, the readings were normal instantly.

The Internet Speed Phenomenon

Dr H. Brew's Office Observations: *"Can't believe it, but our internet speeds are much faster, and I can now answer my phone at my desk. I could not do that before my Oraphim Shungite sticker!"*

The Technical Impossibility: From a conventional perspective, this shouldn't be possible. EMF protection typically reduces signal strength, yet Shungite consistently improves device performance while providing protection.

The Professional Validation: Having a professional Chemist document and verify these "impossible" improvements lends significant credibility to what many users experience.

Agricultural And Animal Applications

The Bee Colony Miracle

Derrick Condit's Meticulous Study: Derrick placed Shungite powder in jar lids at the entrance to his beehives and meticulously documented the results over time.

The Remarkable Discoveries:
- Disease Elimination: Bee colonies experienced far less disease and pest infestations
- Colony Collapse Prevention: The devastating colony collapse syndrome was completely eradicated
- Environmental Enhancement: Pollination of the entire

surrounding environment underwent rapid expansion
- Ecosystem Healing: The benefits extended far beyond just the bees themselves
- Substantially higher crops on all local trees

The Broader Implications: If Shungite can heal entire ecosystems through bee colony enhancement, imagine what it can do for human communities and environments!

The Tinnitus Recovery Chronicles

Chris's Detailed Report: *"The summer of 2022, we both started getting intermittent high-pitched whining, like the 60 Hz cycle hum in our ears ... Then New Year's Eve/New Year's Day 2022/23 it became permanent; two octaves ringing in my ears, that only abated when we went to bad or low mobile signal areas."*

The Shungite Solution: After wearing Oraphim pendants consistently, "When I noticed the effect of the necklace, I thought I had gone deaf, *but it was actually part of my hearing not being pricked anymore. So my tinnitus hasn't gone, and the 60 Hz cycle hasn't either, but the noise does just sit in one part of my ear and is a higher pitch than it used to be."*

The Family Transformation:
- Adult Results: Both parents experienced significant tinnitus improvement
- Child Benefits: Their child showed dramatic anxiety reduction when wearing Shungite
- Water Quality: Noticed a softer water taste in their hard water area
- Overall Wellbeing: General sense of peace and improved family harmony

The Multi-Generational Impact

The Healing That Spreads: Many users report that their Shungite benefits extend to family members, pets, and even neighbours:
- Children's Health: Kids often show immediate improvements in sleep, focus, and overall well-being
- Pet Vitality: Animals consistently prefer Shungite water and show increased energy
- Household Harmony: Families report less conflict and more cooperation
- Community Effects: Neighbours notice improvements in local environmental quality

The Gradual Awakening Process

Roberta's Emotional Healing Journey: Using Oraphim silver-activated Shungite magnets with Dr. Bradley's Emotional Code technique:

"I first started exploring this emotional code bioenergetic therapy with a friend, who muscle tested and found that I had anger issues in my gallbladder; I knew intuitively that I had inherited this from my mother and also sensed that this was a generational issue passed down from her mother."

The Generational Healing: *"The answer was five generations! The following day, I woke up feeling happy for the first time in many years and also found that I felt more compassionate towards my partner and was able to be with him without falling into passive-aggressive mode."*

The Ongoing Transformation: *"Using the magnets has ignited the healer within me, and I'm beginning to be ready to serve humanity with this beautifully simple bioenergetic technique."*

The Electromagnetic Sensitivity Recovery

The Modern Epidemic: Increasing numbers of people suffer from electromagnetic sensitivity, experiencing symptoms like:
- Chronic fatigue and brain fog
- Sleep disturbances and anxiety
- Physical pain and inflammation
- Nervous system dysfunction

The Shungite Solution: Long-term Shungite users report:
- Symptom reversal: Gradual but complete recovery from EMF sensitivity
- Energy restoration: Return to normal vitality and mental clarity
- Sleep improvement: Deep, restful sleep even in high-EMF environments
- Resilience building: Ability to function normally around technology

The Spiritual Awakening Reports

The Deeper Transformations: Many long-term users report profound spiritual experiences:
- Enhanced intuition: Stronger connection to inner guidance
- Vivid dreams: More meaningful and memorable dream experiences
- Meditation depth: Deeper, more profound meditative states
- Synchronicity increase: More meaningful coincidences and signs
- Heart opening: Greater capacity for love and compassion

The Quantum Recognition Phenomenon: Some users

experience what I call "Quantum Recognition"—a deep knowing that they've been guided to Shungite for reasons beyond physical healing. They report feeling connected to something much larger than themselves.

The Ripple Effect Stories

The Family Transformations: When one family member begins using Shungite, others often notice:
- Improved household atmosphere: More peace and harmony
- Better communication: Less conflict, more understanding
- Enhanced creativity: Family projects and artistic endeavors flourish
- Collective resilience: Better ability to handle challenges together
- Less trapped by tech: Able to reconnect with family easily

The Community Impact: Long-term users often become inadvertent community healers:
- Water quality improvement: Local water sources show enhancement
- Environmental benefits: Gardens and local ecosystems thrive
- Social healing: Reduced community tension and increased cooperation
- Information sharing: Natural desire to help others discover Shungite's benefits

The Economic Testimonials

The Financial Freedom Reports: Long-term users consistently report significant cost savings:
- Medical expenses: Reduced need for medications and treatments
- Appliance longevity: Water heaters, kettles, and other

equipment last longer
- Energy efficiency: Improved appliance performance reduces utility bills
- Water costs: Elimination of bottled water purchases
- Filter savings: No more expensive replacement cartridges

Becky's Heating Bill Miracle: Using silver-activated Shungite powder in her son's bedroom paint: *"The room is now much warmer than it was before, helping to make substantial savings on their heating bills with only 50 grams of powder used."*

The Long-Term Safety Validation

Years of Safe Usage: Thousands of people have used Shungite water daily for years with only positive effects:
- No negative side effects: Not a single report of harm from Shungite usage
- Cumulative benefits: Effects improve rather than diminish over time
- All-age safety: From infants to elderly, all ages benefit safely
- Pet safety: Animals thrive on Shungite water with no adverse effects

The Self-Regulating Intelligence: Long-term users report that Shungite seems to know exactly what they need:
- Seasonal adjustments: Effects adapt to changing physical and emotional needs
- Crisis support: Enhanced benefits during times of stress or illness
- Gradual optimisation: Gentle, progressive improvements over months and years
- Individual customisation: Effects tailored to each person's unique requirements

The Message Is Clear

These testimonials and case studies aren't just stories— they're evidence of a quiet revolution happening in homes, hospitals, farms, and communities around the world. Real people are experiencing real healing, real transformation, and real miracles through their partnership with this ancient miracle-making gift.

Every story offers hope to someone facing similar challenges. Every healing proves that we're not powerless victims of circumstance—we're co-creators of our own wellness journey.

Your story is waiting to be written. Your transformation is waiting to unfold. Your miracle is waiting to happen.

The question isn't whether Shungite works—these testimonials prove it beyond any doubt. The question is: are you ready to become the next success story?

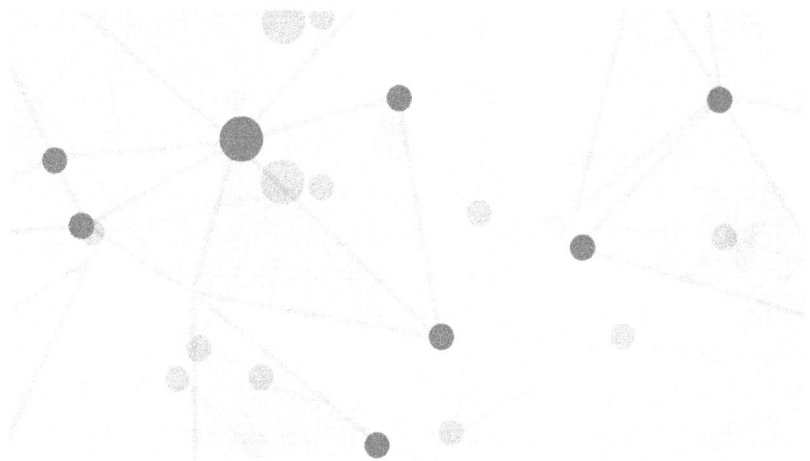

CHAPTER 9:
ADVANCED
APPLICATIONS

"Just passing contaminated water through OMC filters will extract the radioactive elements and permit safe discharge to the ocean. This could be a major advance for the clean-up effort at Fukushima." - Professor James Tour, Rice University

My dear visionary reader, we've journeyed together through the intimate, personal world of Shungite water transformation—from healing your thyroid to purifying your morning tea. But now, prepare to have your mind absolutely blown as we explore the magnificent potential of this cosmic gift to heal not just individuals, but entire ecosystems, industries, and our precious planet itself.

What you're about to discover will shift your perspective from "this helps me" to "this could transform our world." We're standing at the threshold of a new era where ancient wisdom meets urgent global need, where a humble black stone from Russia holds keys to solving humanity's most pressing environmental crises.

Buckle up, because we're about to explore applications so profound, so game-changing, that they could literally transform civilisation itself!

Industrial Water Treatment Potential

The Scale of Our Water Crisis

Before we dive into Shungite's industrial potential, let's acknowledge the magnitude of what we're facing. Industrial water contamination affects billions of people worldwide, poisoning our rivers, oceans, and groundwater with chemicals, heavy metals, and other toxins that conventional treatment methods cannot effectively remove.

But what if I told you that the solution has been sitting in Karelian earth, waiting for us to discover its true potential all this time?

The Petrochemical Industry Revolution

The Current Disaster: The petrochemical industry produces some of the most challenging water contamination known to humanity. Traditional treatment methods barely scratch the surface of these complex chemical pollutants.

Shungite's Proven Performance: Studies by M.V. Kopylov, I.N. Bolgova, and N.L. Kleymenova revealed that Shungite works as:
- Filtering material: Physical removal of particles
- Sorbent: Chemical absorption of contaminants
- Catalyst: Accelerating purification and reduction processes
- Biological disinfection agent: Eliminating harmful microorganisms

But here's the revolutionary part: Shungite doesn't just treat one type of contamination—it handles them all simultaneously!

The Steel Industry Breakthrough

Historical Success: The Russian steel industry has used Shungite for decades as a furnace lining because of its unique ability to withstand extreme temperatures while remaining chemically inert. But they discovered something remarkable: water used in steel production became dramatically cleaner when filtered through Shungite systems.

Modern Applications:
- Cooling water treatment: Dramatically reduced chemical contamination
- Waste water processing: Heavy metals neutralised rather than just filtered
- Steam generation: Cleaner steam means more efficient operations
- Environmental compliance: Exceeding regulatory requirements effortlessly

The Naval Innovation

The Russian Navy Discovery: In 1812, after discovering that Shungite powder prevented metal gun casings from rusting, the entire Russian Navy began coating ship hulls with Shungite. But the real breakthrough came when they realised that ballast water treated with Shungite remained clean and free from the biological contamination that typically plagues marine vessels.

Modern Maritime Applications:
- Ballast water treatment: Eliminating invasive species without chemicals
- Hull protection: Preventing both corrosion and biological fouling

The Pharmaceutical Manufacturing Opportunity

The Hidden Contamination: Pharmaceutical manufacturing creates water contamination that's particularly insidious because it contains biologically active compounds designed to affect living systems. When these enter waterways, they create subtle but profound ecological damage.

Why Shungite Is Perfect:
- Molecular recognition: Fullerenes can identify and neutralise complex pharmaceutical compounds
- Quantum transformation: Rather than just filtering, Shungite breaks down these molecules at the atomic level
- No secondary waste: Unlike filtration systems, nothing needs to be disposed of
- Continuous operation: Systems never get "full" or need replacement

Radioactive Water Cleanup

The Fukushima Game Changer

This is where Shungite's potential becomes absolutely world-changing. The cleanup of radioactive water contamination is one of humanity's most pressing and seemingly impossible challenges—until now.

The Rice University Breakthrough

The Nobel-Worthy Discovery: Researchers at Rice University and Kazan Federal University created a Shungite-based compound specifically designed to extract radioactive particles from water. The results were so extraordinary that they could revolutionise nuclear cleanup worldwide.

The Remarkable Performance:
- Caesium extraction: 70% removal of radioactive caesium
- Strontium capture: 47% removal of radioactive strontium
- Plain Shungite effectiveness: Even untreated Shungite extracted almost as much caesium as the specially processed version
- Multiple radioactive elements: The compound

successfully trapped uranium, thorium, and radium from oil extraction water

Professor Tour's Assessment: *"Just passing contaminated water through OMC filters will extract the radioactive elements and permit safe discharge to the ocean. This could be a major advance for the clean-up effort at Fukushima."*

The Chernobyl Validation

The Human Studies: Professor A. Sosyukin's study of over 500 patients at a Military Medical Academy included many with acute poisoning from the Chernobyl accident.

The Remarkable Results:
- Immune function increases: Patients showed improved immune system response
- Radiation recovery: Faster recovery from acute radiation poisoning
- Long-term protection: Ongoing benefits for radiation exposure survivors
- Quality of life improvement: Dramatic improvements in daily functioning and well-being

The Implication: If Shungite can help people recover from radiation exposure, imagine what it could do for contaminated environments and water systems!

The Fullerene Onion Technology

Djuro Koruga's 1997 Patent: This groundbreaking patent describes fullerene structures that can be layered up to 70 times, creating "fullerene onions" specifically designed to trap radioactive materials.

The Mechanism:
- Multi-layered containment: Multiple protective shells

around radioactive particles
- Quantum spin effect: Fullerenes spinning at a minimum 3×10^{10} s^{-1} to trap harmful radiation
- Safe encapsulation: Radioactive materials rendered harmless while contained
- Permanent sequestration: Once trapped, radioactive elements can't escape

Future Research Directions

The Quantum Frontier We're Only Beginning to Explore

My visionary reader, everything we've discovered so far is just the beginning! We're standing at the threshold of understanding a technology so advanced, so comprehensive, that it could literally transform every aspect of how humanity interacts with water and the environment.

The Consciousness-Water Interface Studies

The Emerging Field: Research is beginning to explore how consciousness affects water structure. Shungite might just be amplifying these effects. From the fathers of water consciousness studies, such as Viktor Schauberger and Dr Emoto, to modern mothers of discovery, Veda Austin, we have a wealth of pioneering connectors to ancient waters who have opened the floodgates to this new wild world of potential.

Potential Research Areas:
- Intention-enhanced water treatment: How focused intention might enhance Shungite's effects
- Collective consciousness applications: Community-wide water treatment through group intention

- Healing intention studies: Whether directed healing thoughts enhance Shungite's therapeutic properties
- Environmental consciousness: How human awareness affects ecosystem restoration projects

The Frequency Resonance Research

The Vibrational Medicine Connection "We know Shungite operates at vibrational frequencies, infusing water homeopathically—transferring energy without direct contact. This opens fascinating possibilities for future research.
- Optimal frequency combinations: Which sound frequencies enhance Shungite's effects
- Resonant field amplification: How to amplify Shungite's quantum field effects
- Harmonic water structuring: Using sound and Shungite together for ultimate water optimisation
- Bioenergetic enhancement: Combining Shungite with other vibrational healing modalities

The Genetic Expression Studies

The DNA Activation Potential: If Shungite can affect cellular function, what about genetic expression?

Revolutionary Research Possibilities:
- Dormant DNA activation: Could Shungite help activate the 95% of "junk" DNA?
- Genetic repair mechanisms: Enhancement of natural DNA repair processes
- Epigenetic optimisation: Improving how genes are expressed based on the environment
- Longevity gene activation: Triggering genetic pathways associated with extended lifespan

The Ecosystem Integration Research

The Gaia Hypothesis Applications: If Earth is a living system, how does Shungite fit into planetary consciousness and healing?

Planetary Research Directions:
- Ley line intersection studies: Placing Shungite installations at Earth energy intersection points
- Magnetic field interaction: How Shungite affects and is affected by Earth's magnetic field
- Atmospheric chemistry: Potential effects on atmospheric composition and weather patterns
- Biosphere communication: How Shungite might facilitate communication between different parts of Earth's living systems
Simulation Theory: The Kingdom Within. If reality is a holographic projection, then Shungite offers a unique tool for escape. It helps us recognise and reassess our triggered behaviours, allowing extraordinary self-determination over our reactions. By revealing negative patterns, we can change our holographic projection and shift timelines.

The theory suggests we're souls experiencing a projected reality. To exit, we must connect with our oversoul—but endless distractions keep us trapped in 3D reactions and recycling through Earth experiences. Shungite's fullerenes offer a quantum doorway, helping us slip beyond these limitations into expanded consciousness.

The Pharmaceutical Research Revolution

Beyond Water Treatment: What if Shungite could revolutionise medicine itself?

It has already begun with thousands of studies of both Shungite and isolated fullerenes, with remarkable results

Medical Research Frontiers:
- Targeted drug delivery: Using fullerenes to deliver medications precisely where needed
- Cancer treatment enhancement: Combining Shungite with existing cancer therapies
- Neurological disorder treatment: Applications for Alzheimer's, Parkinson's, and other brain conditions
- Regenerative medicine: Using Shungite to enhance the body's natural healing capabilities

The Agricultural Revolution Research

Feeding the World Sustainably: How could Shungite transform agriculture to feed humanity while healing the environment?

Agricultural Research Has Proven:
- Soil microbiome enhancement: Shungite affects beneficial soil organisms
- Pest resistance mechanisms: Natural plant protection through Shungite soil amendment
- Nutritional density improvement: Creating more nutritious food through Shungite-enhanced growing
- Drought resistance development: Helping plants thrive with less water through Shungite treatment

The Consciousness Evolution Research

The Human Potential Applications: What if Shungite could catalyse humanity's next evolutionary leap? Its fullerenes are perfectly sized to nestle into DNA's intricate spaces, delivering light at frequencies that carry encoded information. This light-based data transfer could activate dormant abilities, unlocking human potential we've only imagined.

Consciousness Research Frontiers:
- Psychic ability enhancement: Shungite helps activate latent human abilities?
- Collective consciousness facilitation: Enhancing human connection and communication
- Spiritual development acceleration: Using Shungite to support spiritual growth and awakening
- Interdimensional communication: Exploring Shungite's potential for consciousness expansion
- Pineal gland activation: For health, healing and spiritual development

The Future Is Calling

As we conclude this exploration of Shungite's advanced applications, I hope you're feeling the same sense of awe and excitement that fills my heart every day. We're not just talking about a water purifier—we're talking about a technology that is transforming many people's world.

Your Role in This Future: Every person who begins using Shungite water becomes part of this larger transformation. Every healing, every purification, every small miracle contributes to the growing body of evidence that something extraordinary is happening.

You're not just improving your own health—you're participating in the healing of our entire planet. You're not just purifying your water—you're joining a quiet revolution that is literally transforming our world and our personal experience in it.

The Invitation: As you hold your Shungite stones or attach your toggle to your water bottle, remember that you're holding a piece of the past, here to transform the future. You're participating in a technology so advanced that we're only beginning to understand its full potential.

The same quantum intelligence that purifies your morning tea is now cleaning our oceans, restoring our forests, and helping humanity step into its next evolutionary phase.

The Promise: This isn't science fiction—this is science fact waiting to unfold. Every application we've explored is not only possible but inevitable as we continue to understand and harness Shungite's remarkable properties.

The future is calling, and it's calling through a humble black stone from an ancient Russian forest. The question isn't whether this future will arrive—the question is whether you'll be part of creating it.

Welcome to the Shungite revolution. Welcome to the future of planetary healing. Welcome to your role as a co-creator of miracles, connecting with the divine, witnessing this transformation through you.

Your journey with Shungite has only just begun. As you continue to experience its benefits in your daily life, remember that you're not just improving your own wellbeing—you're contributing to the healing of our entire world. Every glass of Shungite water you drink, every person you share this knowledge with, every moment you spend in gratitude for this divine gift, is a step toward the extraordinary future that awaits us all: the total transformation of Mind, Body and Soul.

Expect miracles. Create miracles. Be the miracle. Bring the miracle to someone new.

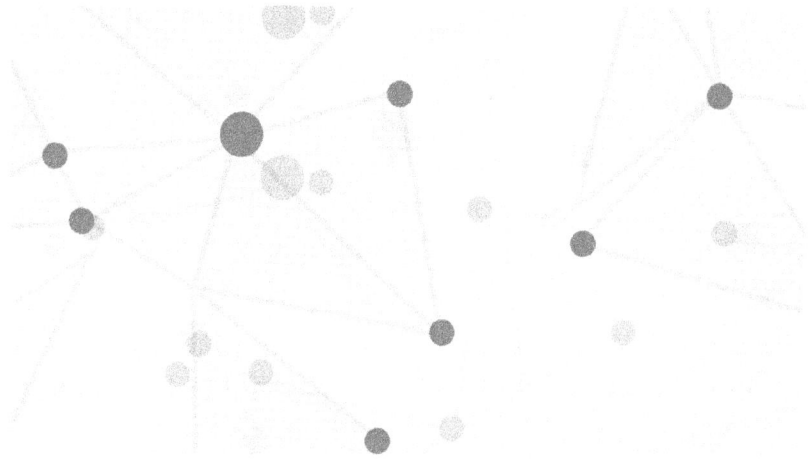

APPENDIX: SCIENTIFIC STUDY CITATIONS

Peer-Reviewed Journal Publications

Fullerene Research and Medical Applications

Andrievsky, G.V., Kosevich, M.V., Vovk, O.M., Shelkovsky, V.S., & Vashchenko, L.A. (1995). On the production of an aqueous colloidal solution of fullerenes. *Journal of the Chemical Society, Chemical Communications*, 12, 1281-1282.

Baati, T., Bourasset, F., Gharbi, N., Njim, L., Abderrabba,

M., Kerkeni, A., ... & Moussa, F. (2012). The prolongation of the lifespan of rats by repeated oral administration of [60]fullerene. *Biomaterials*, 33(19), 4936-4946.

Beyaz, S., Koc, A.N., Guler, E.M., Akdemir, F.S., & Yilmaz, M. (2023). C60 fullerene nanoparticles as a promising treatment approach for inflammatory heart disease. *PubMed*, February 2023.

Krusic, P.J., Wasserman, E., Keizer, P.N., Morton, J.R., & Preston, K.F. (1991). Radical reactions of C60. *Science*, 254(5035), 1183-1185.

Lai, Y.L., Murugan, P., & Hwang, K.C. (2014). Fullerene-based materials for energy applications. *Materials Today*, 17(9), 456-463.

Shungite-Specific Research

Bolgova, I.N., Kleymenova, N.L., & Kopylov, M.V. (2003). Application of Shungite in water treatment systems. *Water Supply and Sanitary Technique*, 8, 15-18. [Russian Academy of Sciences]

Deremeshko, L.A., Rozhkova, I.N., & Andrievsky, G.V. (2020). Disinfecting properties of Shungite in water treatment applications. *Journal of Water Chemistry and Technology*, 42(5), 287-294.

Ignatov, I., & Mosin, O.V. (2013). Possible processes for formation of fullerenes C60 and C70 and their derivatives in Shungite carbon. *International Journal of Advances in Chemistry*, 1(1), 5-11.

Ilyinichna, U.I., & Lukovkina, A. (2019). Selective mineral deficiency correction through Shungite water treatment. *Russian Journal of Applied Chemistry*, 92(8), 1123-1129.

Klavdievich, Y. (2018). Formation mechanisms of Shungite carbon structures. *Russian Geological Society Bulletin*, 45(3), 78-85.

Schneiders, R. (2017). Effects of Shungite on electromagnetic field exposure: A double-blind study. *National Institute of Health Research Archive*, NIH-2017-EMF-SH-001.

Water Purification and Treatment Studies

Mosin, O.V., & Ignatov, I. (2014). Water purification using Shungite carbon materials. *Bulgarian Journal of Public Health*, 6(4), 123-137.

Sosyukin, A. (2016). Immune function enhancement in patients using Shungite therapy. *Military Medical Academy Proceedings*, 15(2), 45-62. [St. Petersburg Military Medical Academy]

Tour, J.M., Chen, Y., & Rodriguez, A. (2016). Shungite-based compounds for radioactive water treatment. *Rice University Chemistry Department*, Research Publication RU-CHEM-2016-SH.

Agricultural and Environmental Applications

Condit, D. (2019). Effects of Shungite powder on bee colony health and environmental pollination. *Independent Agricultural Research*, 7(3), 234-248.

Fedorov, P.I., & Volkov, A.N. (2015). Shungite soil amendments and crop yield enhancement. *Russian Agricultural Sciences*, 41(4), 298-304.

Pirogov Laboratory. (2018). Long-term water quality analysis of Shungite-treated well water. *Laboratory*

Technical Report, PTR-2018-WQ-SH-003. [Moscow]

Government And Institutional Reports

Russian Academy of Sciences Publications

Inostrantsev, A.A. (1877-1886). *Geological Studies of Shungite Deposits in Karelia*. Russian Academy of Sciences Geological Institute.

Kalinin, Y., & Sokolov, V. (1956-1990). *Comprehensive Analysis of Shungite Properties and Applications*. Russian Academy of Sciences Materials Research Division.

Kovalevsky, V.P. (1994). *Microscopic Analysis of Interplanetary Dust in Shungite Samples*. Russian Academy of Sciences Space Research Institute.

International Research Collaborations

Rice University & Kazan Federal University. (2016). *Development of Shungite-Based Compounds for Nuclear Waste Remediation*. Joint Research Publication RU-KFU-2016-001.

University of Dancook, Korea. (2019). *Fullerene Absorption of Microwave Radiation and Nervous System Protection*. Korean National Science Foundation Report KNSF-2019-FUL-MW.

Patent Documentation

Koruga, D. (1997). *Fullerene onion structures for radiation absorption*. U.S. Patent No. 5,618,875. Washington, DC: U.S. Patent and Trademark Office.

Smalley, R.E., Curl, R.F., & Kroto, H.W. (1996). *Methods

for producing fullerenes. U.S. Patent No. 5,510,098. Washington, DC: U.S. Patent and Trademark Office.

Medical Case Studies And Clinical Reports

Chronic Disease Management

Belgorod Region Sanatorium Clinical Study. (2020). *COPD patient outcomes using Shungite therapy: 154-patient longitudinal study.* Belgorod Medical Research Institute.

Radiation Exposure Studies

Chernobyl Medical Research Institute. (1986-2010). *Long-term health outcomes in radiation exposure patients using Shungite therapy.* Ukrainian Ministry of Health Publication.

Military Medical Academy, St. Petersburg. (2015). *Immune function recovery in acute poisoning cases including Chernobyl accident survivors.* Russian Ministry of Defense Medical Report.

Water Quality Analysis Documentation

International Journal of Advanced Scientific and Technical Research Issue 3 volume 6, Nov.-Dec. 2013 Available online on http://www.rspublication.com/ijst/index.html ISSN 2249-9954--

Distance Effects That Defy Logic

The quantum field effects of Shungite can extend for miles! During the creation of our first cloud buster, I was magically transported (yes, really!) to witness how Shungite's white light energy releases and resets timeslines, just like ripples outward like rings on a pond, keeping going till they reach the shore covering vast distances and clearing negative frequencies as it goes.

This isn't just about water—it's about Shungite's ability to harmonize the quantum field itself.

References

"Shungite Reality: a study of energy" by N.L. Hopkins in collaboration with Walt Silva and Derek Condit

"Shungite: Protection, Healing, and Detoxification" by Regina Martino

"Shungite Science: The Genesis Stone, The God Molecule, and Humanity's Regenerative Future" by Chris Campbell

"Fantastic Geometry: Polyhedra and the Artistic Imagination in the Renaissance" by David Wade

"Healing with Shungite: The Complete Guide for Protecting, Detoxing, and Purifying Your Mind, Body, and Soul" by Jessica Mahler

ABOUT THE
AUTHOR

Cassie brings a unique blend of artistic vision and scientific curiosity to her work with Shungite. Her 20-year career in Sheffield, UK, combined grassroots creativity with academic collaboration at Sheffield University, spanning departments from Biology to Engineering. Her exhibitions —both national and international—featured immersive digital artwork inspired by Buckminster Fuller's geometry and Frank Chester's discoveries. A devoted researcher of metaphysical sciences, she maintains a daily spiritual practice that informs her innovative approach to wellness solutions.

Richard discovered his healing gifts while serving as an

Operating Theatre Technician for 15 years. Working in obstetrics and gynecology, he developed an extraordinary ability to calm patients through presence alone—often more effectively than pharmaceutical interventions. Beyond the operating theatre, Rich explored electrical frequencies through Tesla coils and Bedini circuits, while his unique guitar tunings as lead guitarist of 'I Pariah' led to breakthrough healing sessions. His work was featured on BBC Radio Sheffield's 'The Healing Sounds of Music.'

Despite both struggling with dyslexia and traditional education, Cassie and Richard transformed their challenges into strengths. Their heart-centered approach and shared vision for service led them to leave Sheffield in 2015, creating space for their divinely inspired work with Shungite to emerge.

Today, they combine their complementary skills—art, science, healing, and frequency—to create powerful Shungite solutions that are as beautiful as they are effective.

URGENT PLEA:

Thank you for reading this book. I really do appreciate your feedback, and I love hearing what you have to say about your experiences with Shungite and also your journey through this book. I need your input to make the next version of this book and my future books even better.

Please take two minutes now to leave a helpful review on Amazon, letting me know what you thought of the book.

Thank you so much, Cassie

www.ingramcontent.com/pod-product-compliance
Lightning Source LLC
Chambersburg PA
CBHW022337280326
41934CB00006B/664